T0306050

Coaching for Person-Centred Healthcare

This guide introduces a humanistic, solution-focused coaching model, using lived experience to demonstrate how profound changes in our healthcare experiences and system, for patients and staff, are possible; while also supporting readers to develop their own coaching skills.

Combining research, theory, and practice shared through personal experience, readers are introduced to solution-focused, dialogic tools for use in promoting person-centred care. The first section of the book introduces the coaching model and explores its theoretical and philosophical underpinnings, drawing on theories from neuroscience, neurobiology, communication sciences, humanistic psychology, and positive psychology. The second section of the book transitions from theory and research into clinical practice, making evident the broad range of healthcare contexts and domains in which the humanistic, solution-focused approaches are implemented, as well as the profound personal and professional implications associated with their use. The third section of the book focuses on the lived experience of four people, focusing on their interactions with healthcare before and after their coaching training, emphasizing the difference a humanistic, solution-focused approach has made for them and their families.

The final section then turns to organizational change and explores how solution-focused coaching provides insights, perspectives, and aspirations for system change. This engaging text is ideal reading for healthcare professionals, teachers, and leaders looking to develop and improve the care they deliver, the experiences of the people they are working with, and the organizations they deliver it within.

Dr Elaine Cook is the Manager Humanistic Education & Training at Holland Bloorview Kids Rehabilitation Hospital. Her research focus is the neuroscience of optimal functioning and language.

Dr Gilbert J. Greene is Professor Emeritus at The Ohio State University in the College of Social Work.

Joanne Maxwell, PhD (candidate), is Vice President, Experience, Transformation and Social Accountability at Holland Bloorview Kids Rehabilitation Hospital. Her research interests include transitions in care, and client- and family-centred care.

Coaching for Person-Centred Healthcare

A Solution-Focused Approach to Collaborative Care

Edited by Elaine Cook, Gilbert J. Greene, and Joanne Maxwell

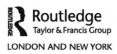

Routledge
Taylor & Francis Group

LONDON AND NEW YORK

Cover credit: Holland Bloorview Humanistic Education & Training

First published 2025
by Routledge
4 Park Square, Milton Park, Abingdon, Oxon OX14 4RN

and by Routledge
605 Third Avenue, New York, NY 10158

Routledge is an imprint of the Taylor & Francis Group, an informa business

British Library Cataloguing-in-Publication Data
A catalogue record for this book is available from the British Library

Library of Congress Cataloging-in-Publication Data
Names: Cook, Elaine (Certified solution-focused coach), editor. |
Greene, Gilbert J., editor. | Maxwell, Joanne, editor.
Title: Coaching for person-centred healthcare : a solution-focused
approach to collaborative care/edited by Elaine Cook, Gilbert Greene,
and Joanne Maxwell.
Description: Abingdon, Oxon; New York, NY : Routledge, 2025. | Includes
bibliographical references and index.
Identifiers: LCCN 2024026463 (print) | LCCN 2024026464 (ebook) | ISBN
9781032539607 (hbk) | ISBN 9781032539560 (pbk) | ISBN
9781003414490 (ebk)
Subjects: MESH: Patient-Centered Care | Mentoring | Patient Care Team |
Professional-Patient Relations
Classification: LCC RA425 (print) | LCC RA425 (ebook) | NLM W 18 |
DDC 362.1--dc23/eng/20240618
LC record available at https://lccn.loc.gov/2024026463
LC ebook record available at https://lccn.loc.gov/2024026464

ISBN: 978-1-032-53960-7 (hbk)
ISBN: 978-1-032-53956-0 (pbk)
ISBN: 978-1-003-41449-0 (ebk)

DOI: 10.4324/9781003414490

Typeset in Times New Roman
by KnowledgeWorks Global Ltd.

Contents

Contributors

Dr Laura R. Bowman (formerly Hartman), PhD, OT Reg. (Ont.), is the Project Manager for Research & Evaluation, Employment Pathways, at Holland Bloorview Kids Rehabilitation Hospital.

Jacqueline Carver, MSW, LISW, is the Clinical Director of Mental and Behavioral Health Outreach Services Area Agency on Aging, in Lima, Ohio, USA.

Brian Freel is a Solution-Focused Health Care Coach as well as a Collaborative Behaviour Support Coach & Program Facilitator at Holland Bloorview Kids Rehabilitation Hospital.

Nikky Henderson is the Program Assistant for the Humanistic Education and Training Team at Holland Bloorview Kids Rehabilitation Hospital.

Amy Hu, BScPhm, MHA, CHE, is a Quality Improvement (QI) professional with a background in clinical pharmacy. Amy uses solution-focused communication principles to engage leaders and staff throughout the organization. Amy is committed to staff psychological safety and well-being as the foundation to achieve operational excellence in healthcare.

Sarah Keenan, MPH, CSFC, PCC, is an Organization Development (OD) professional working in healthcare. Sarah has clinical, teaching, and research experience, all in the healthcare system. Sarah uses a solution-focused approach to support positive shifts in workplace culture, and support healthcare leadership development.

Wesley Magee-Saxton is an actor as well as a Collaborative Behaviour Support Coach at Holland Bloorview Kids Rehabilitation Hospital.

Dolly Menna-Dack, MHSc, is Senior Bioethicist and Interim Senior Director of Collaborative Practice at Holland Bloorview Kids Rehabilitation Hospital.

Candace Muskat is Family Mentor at Holland Bloorview Kids Rehabilitation Hospital as well as a Solution-Focused Health Care Coach in private practice.

Amanda Kelly Mai York Quan Musto works in the early learning and development department at Holland Bloorview Kids Rehabilitation Hospital.

Moira Peña, OT Reg. (Ont.), is Team Lead, Autism Projects & Programs at Holland Bloorview Kids Rehabilitation Hospital, as well as a Lecturer, Adjunct Appointment, University of Toronto Department of Occupational Science & Occupational Therapy.

Cathy Petta is a Registered Nurse, Certified Solution-Focused Health Care Coach and Facilitator at Holland Bloorview Kids Rehabilitation Hospital.

Dr Heidi Schwellnus is a Collaborative Practice Leader at Holland Bloorview Kids Rehabilitation Hospital. Her areas of research include solution-focused coaching in healthcare and childhood resilience.

Gunjan Seth is a Family Mentor at Holland Bloorview Kids Rehabilitation Hospital.

Anna Trbovich is a mum to two lovely boys. She is also a lawyer. She has a Bachelor of Kinesiology from Acadia University, a Bachelor of Laws from the University of New Brunswick, and a Master of Laws from Harvard.

Kim Weishar is Superintendent of Program Services at Simcoe Muskoka Catholic District School Board, in Ontario, Canada.

Acknowledgements

This book could not have become a reality without the support and contributions of many people. First, we want to thank Grace McInnes, Health and Social Care Publisher at Routledge/Taylor & Francis Group, for her ongoing enthusiastic support for this project, and the invaluable help of Madii Cherry-Moreton, assistant editor also at Routledge/Taylor & Francis Group. Next, we want to thank all the other chapter authors in this book. We appreciate their hard work and willingness to share their stories of the humanistic, solution-focused journeys. We also want to acknowledge the valuable assistance of Nikky Henderson, Program Assistant, Solution-Focused Practice in the Humanistic Education and Training Program at Holland Bloorview Kids Rehabilitation Hospital, who has been in her position from the beginning of the program and also contributed a chapter to this book.

Elaine Cook

I would like to acknowledge two people who I feel have helped guide me to this place in my journey, a journey towards my best self. First, Haesun Moon, who is responsible for my love affair with solution-focused practice; I watch her with wonder and awe. Second, Joanne Maxwell, co-editor of this book, and my manager. Joanne has held a vision for healthcare that few leaders have, she has provided unwavering support for our bold growth, and provided the autonomy I needed to lead it.

Gilbert "Gil" Greene

I am thankful for the invaluable conversations I have had over the years with many talented clinicians, especially Mo Yee Lee, PhD, Professor and Director of the PhD Program at The Ohio State University College of Social Work; Pamela Scott, PhD, LISW-S, Director of Clinical Development, The Buckeye Ranch, Columbus, Ohio; Susan Saltzburg, PhD, Associate Professor Emeritus, The Ohio State University, College of Social Work; and Matthew Selekman, LCSW, Director of Partners for Collaborative Solutions, Evanston, Illinois. These conversations have deepened my appreciation for and understanding of the importance of focusing on identifying, amplifying, and reinforcing client strengths, competencies, and resources. Let's continue the conversations!

Joanne Maxwell

I am incredibly grateful for the many colleagues, clinicians, researchers, and clients and families that have helped me to appreciate and recognize the incredible power of solution-focused practice. Our work in building capacity in solution-focused practice is about so much more than learning a clinical skill. It is a means of creating engagement, fostering agency, and deepening relationships. I feel especially thankful for the role Elaine Cook has played in my solution-focused journey. Her endless enthusiasm for and commitment to this work is undeniable and positively infectious.

Foreword

In a world increasingly dominated by technology and artificial intelligence, the primal need for human connection and empathy in professional practice has become more vital than ever. As a communication scientist and a proponent of solution-focused methodologies, I have consistently advocated approaches that prioritize the human element, emphasizing relational and dialogic processes. It is against this backdrop that *Coaching for Person-Centred Healthcare: A Solution-Focused Approach to Collaborative Care* arrives as a timely and significant contribution to the discourse on humanistic care, highlighting the enduring importance of this approach.

This book is more than a collection of chapters; it is a celebration of an approach that has profoundly impacted lives across various walks and waves. It serves as a tribute to the multiple scenes of solution-focused practices, unfolding in settings that range from research and reflection to hands-on practices. By showcasing the application of solution-focused practices in these varied environments, this volume highlights the versatility and adaptability of this approach. What makes this book particularly special is its holistic embrace of care. It extends much-needed attention not only to patients, students, and clients, but also to the carers themselves – the clinicians, parents, educators, and practitioners. It serves as a poignant reminder of the importance of caring for those who dedicate their lives to caring for others. Solution-focused practice serves as a modality of this care, while the person-centred perspective upholds the multiplicity of our unique needs and wants.

One of the most evocative aspects of this book is its exploration of lived experiences that transcend the tribulations and trials of being human. These narratives capture the heart of solution-focused practice, showcasing its power to facilitate healing and curate stories of purpose, possibilities, and progress. The cascading effect of these personal transformations on larger systems emphasizes the ripple effects of bringing "cura" – healing – back into the forefront of our work.

As you journey through the pages of this book, I invite you to embrace the warmth and wisdom contained within. Let the stories and insights inspire you to integrate these humanistic and solution-focused principles into your practice, contributing to a more compassionate and empathetic world. May this book serve as a guide, a source of inspiration, and a reminder of the profound impact we can have when we centre our work around the human spirit.

With heartfelt gratitude and admiration for the heroes in the field,

Haesun Moon, PhD
Toronto, Canada

Section One

Theory and Practice

1 Healing Healthcare

How Coaching Leads to Optimal Functioning for Clients and Staff

Elaine Cook

Headlines all over the world are issuing dire warnings about the state of healthcare in their respective countries. For example: in the UK, *Why is Britain's health service, a much-loved national treasure, falling apart?* (Edwards, 2023); in Canada, *Health care is showing the cracks it's had for decades. Why it will take more than cash to fix it* (Brend, 2022); in the US, *Doctors aren't burned out from overwork. We're demoralized by our health system* (Reinhart, 2023); in Asia, *Healthcare workers are at their breaking point but most don't want to quit* (Leng, 2022); in Australia, *Why Australia needs a systemic response to burnout* (Warby, 2022); and, in Europe, *The health workforce crisis in Europe is no longer a looming threat – it is here and now* (WHO, 2023). Also strikingly similar is the almost universal acknowledgement that burnout among healthcare providers – which is a factor that diminishes care – has never been higher (Berg, 2022; McEvoy & Thompson, 2022). There are as many hypotheses as there are headlines about the reasons for the healthcare crisis that many are experiencing. Researchers suggest, however, that the current deficit-based, hierarchal medical model, a model that conditions our clients/patients to be passive and compliant users of the system (Haus, 2017; Rider et al., 2018), as well as the emphasis on economic and commercial metrics that are incongruent with personal and healthcare values (Rider et al., 2018), has contributed to a dissonance that is negatively impacting healthcare around the world.

Coaching for Change

System renewal and repair requires a profound shift in the status quo. At Holland Bloorview Kids Rehabilitation Hospital, Canada's largest paediatric rehabilitation hospital, we have provided coaching education and training to over 2,500 clinicians in the past two years. All client-facing staff are required to attend four half days of training, which is offered, along with one-on-one coaching support, as part of the onboarding process. Additionally, collaborative behaviour support coaches are available five days a week to support staff in situ when challenging behaviours occur or are expected to occur, and if that isn't enough, we provide coaching classes to parents as well as youth leaders. To buttress all these initiatives, we created a year-long, externally certificated course (Certified Solution-focused Health Care Coach, CSF-HCC) that is offered to internal staff for free and externals

DOI: 10.4324/9781003414490-2

at a cost. This is in addition to a suite of half-day, topic-specific coaching work-shops that are offered monthly on a rotating basis, internally and externally. The certificate course is delivered in a manner that embeds learning into the work day of our clinicians, which ensures their learning is context-specific and not perceived as something "extra" that is required. The investment in these initiatives has paid off in multiple ways, the most obvious perhaps being the chapters in this book, where graduates of the certificate program share their personal and lived experi-ence of change, transformation and optimal functioning. All of this reinforces evi-dence suggesting that coaching improves satisfaction and outcomes for healthcare providers (Manzi et al., 2017; Palamara et al., 2015; Seko et al., 2020; Wolff et al., 2020), as well as improves outcomes for patients and families (Boehmer et al., 2016; Dubé et al., 2015; King, 2019; Maini et al., 2020; Schwellnus et al., 2015).

More broadly, the value of coaching in healthcare has been identified in many diverse healthcare contexts, including: medical student training amplified person-centered care (Maini et al., 2020); decreased physician and staff burnout and emotional exhaustion (Dyrbye et al., 2019; MacLeod et al., 2017; Palamara et al., 2015); organizational development (Abington, 2013, King et al., 2021; Seko et al., 2020; Zulman et al., 2020); and increased mental health and protective neural networks (Marano et al., 2021). Yet, despite all the good news associated with coaching outcomes in healthcare, we noticed early in our program's development that our coaching model (known as solution-focused coaching) wasn't enough for clinicians and physicians from various disciplines, who were endeavouring to en-gage and collaborate with clients and families who were often emotional and/or escalated. They needed and wanted an evidenced-based framework to guide their understanding of client responses and behaviours, as well as guide their dialogic strategies in a way that operationalized the humanistic principles of our program. Over a period of two years and two different cohorts, the Funnel of Optimal Func-tioning (FOF; Cook, 2022) was developed as that educational tool. The model is founded on principles and theory of optimal functioning, as well as the neurosci-ence and neurobiology of language. However, before describing the FOF in more detail, it is essential that we distinguish the toolbox from the tool.

Building the Toolbox

We noticed an interesting phenomenon with healthcare learners early in our educa-tion and training journey. With a room full of clinicians, therapists, advocates and administrators, we'd begin by asking a version of the very traditional solution-focused "best hopes" question, "How might you know, at the end of our time to-gether, that it has been helpful or useful for you?" Without fail, the most common answer was (and still is) generally, *tools for our toolbox*. This might not be surpris-ing considering the context; a group of incredibly busy people who want to learn and then get on with their jobs. Succumbing to this demand, although easy and therefore tempting, is a mistake and a contributing factor to gaps in continuing edu-cation for healthcare providers. Researchers reveal that motivation and emotional factors are cited as barriers (Reis et al., 2022; Surr et al., 2020) to education and training programs, and simply providing learners with tools is neither motivating, nor does it provide an emotional connection. This explains the reaction when I ask learners to tell me about their toolbox and how these particular tools will fit in that toolbox. There is nothing more important to a tradesperson than their toolbox. It is a home for their tools, it helps them find a particular tool when needed, it keeps their work organized and therefore helps them to do their job more effectively. As educators and trainers, we need to *first* help learners build a toolbox – a framework for organizing their tools, so they are not only emotionally connected to those tools, but they are also motivated to use them and can find them when needed.

Our Funnel of Optional Functioning (FOF) and solution-focused, dialogic tools are kept in a humanistic toolbox that enables practitioners to experience consonance between healthcare practice as well as professional and personal values. Researchers suggest that dissonance between professional and health system values contributes to burnout (Rider et al., 2018). A humanistic perspective invites care

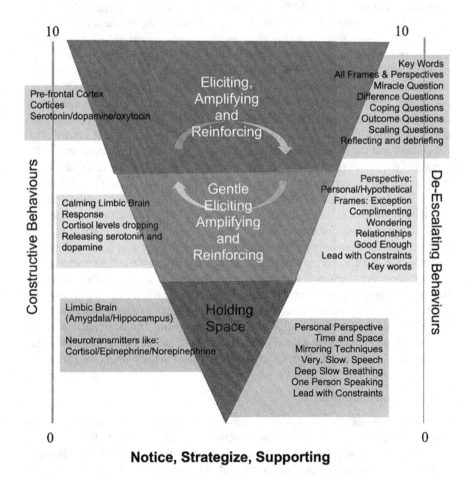

Figure 1.1 The Funnel of Optimal Functioning

providers to become collaborators instead of experts (van den Goor et al., 2020); to adopt a dialogical healing approach as opposed to a transactional fixing approach (Agarwal, 2020; Kumagai et al., 2018; Remen, 1999); and to see their clients as whole, instead of broken (Schneider et al., 2001). A humanistic approach illuminates the client's inherent strengths and resources (Rogers, 1979) as opposed to the deficit focus currently enshrined in healthcare (Haus, 2017). The consonance and congruency of a healthcare practice grounded in principles of humanism motivates and provides an emotional resonance for healthcare providers, which can then be operationalized with tools and skills. These tools and skills now have a home.

As mentioned, the FOF was created as a coaching tool for clinicians and healthcare professionals learning to facilitate humanistic, coaching conversations with their clients and families. It provides a framework that helps practitioners to better understand their clients' behaviours and emotions and the coaching interventions that best support optimal functioning in that particular moment in time. The funnel represents the human brain. At the bottom of the funnel (Holding Space Zone), one is primarily functioning from the limbic or emotional brain. At the top of the funnel (Eliciting, Amplifying and Reinforcing Zone), one is using their whole brain and the pre-frontal cortex is fully engaged. On the left side of the funnel are the neurobiological indicators for each zone and on the right side are the dialogic and coaching skills/tools that can be used to engage the client in each zone, while aiming to help them move up the funnel towards optimal functioning. On either side of the funnel are two scales which provide coaches with an assessment guide. Both scales are high, 10 (optimal functioning) to low, 0. The left scale is constructive behaviours and the right scale is de-escalating behaviours, which mean that at the bottom of the scales (0) there are no constructive behaviours and escalation is high, while at the top of both scales constructive behaviours are maximized and the individual is fully de-escalated. Therefore, once the clinician assesses where the client might be on the funnel (using the 10–0 scales), there is an immediate understanding of what is happening for the client (and themselves) from a neurobiological perspective and the most appropriate strategies to engage the client given that understanding. We call the process Noticing, Strategizing, Supporting. First, the clinician notices where the client might be on the funnel (using the scales and the left side of the funnel), then they strategize (Holding Space; Gentle Eliciting, Amplifying, Reinforcing; Eliciting, Amplifying, Reinforcing), and finally they support the client using the skills and tools that align with their assessment. The Noticing, Strategizing, Supporting table is the funnel in table form with detailed descriptions of what the clinician might notice about the client at each zone in the funnel (see Table 1.1).

Optimal Functioning

A secondary benefit of the funnel is the implicit goal of the clinician-coach to amplify the client's optimal functioning (OF) – regardless of any other therapeutic intervention required by the clinician – by facilitating a conversation/dialogue that helps the client to move up the funnel. As the client's optimal functioning is enhanced, their health outcomes improve (Diener et al., 2017) as well as their

Table 1.1 What to Notice Behaviour Inventory

Holding Space	Gentle Eliciting, Amplifying and Reinforcing	Eliciting, Amplifying and Reinforcing
Visual (physical cues)	**Visual (physical cues)**	**Visual (physical cues)**
• staring straight at staff and hardly blinking • eyebrows pulled down, upper eyelids pulled up, lower eyelids pulled up, margins of lips rolled in, lips may be tightened • red face • breathing rapidly • stiff shoulders • clinched fist • in staff's personal space	• infrequent eye contact • inner corners of eyebrows raised, eyelids loose, lip corners pulled down • habitually turning away from staff • change in body posture • change in body tension • change in communication style • change in attitude • change in receptiveness • change in emotional awareness	• sustained eye contact • muscle around the eyes tightened, "crows feet" wrinkles around the eyes, cheeks raised, lip corners raised upwards • facing full body towards staff • comfortable body position • social/emotional repertoire is broad and constructive • receptive • engaged
Auditory and Verbal	**Auditory and Verbal**	**Auditory and Verbal**
• talking fast • yelling • responds to staff too quickly or not at all • questioning, challenging or threatening staff • using foul or inappropriate language	• slow rate of speech • low volume of speech • unresponsive or delayed responses to staff • short or abbreviated responses to staff	• relaxed and sometimes rapid rate of speech • varying volumes • appropriate and timely responses to staff • lengthy and sometimes expanding responses to staff
Physical		
• harm to self, others or property		

therapeutic goals (King et al., 2017). We can make these assertions thanks to robust research in the fields of positive psychology (PP) and neuroscience.

First, PP research confirms that when the strengths of individuals are emphasized, their subjective well-being is amplified and this contributes to optimal functioning (van Nieuwerburgh & Oades, 2017). PP is considered by many as the research of optimal functioning, which is often referred to as subjective well-being (Green et al., 2006; Green & Palmer, 2018; Linley et al., 2006). Although subjective well-being may be considered more ambiguous than researchers prefer, there is consensus around factors that influence well-being and optimal functioning: agency, resilience, optimism, engagement, positive emotions and self-esteem (Dolcos et al., 2020; Kibe & Boniwell, 2015; Lyubomirsky et al., 2006; Nafstad, 2015).

From a neuroscience perspective, recent research, with the help of brain imaging, has greatly improved our knowledge and understanding about contributing factors related to well-being and optimal functioning (King, 2019). Through the

study of patterns of electrical and chemical activity in our brains, associations between thoughts, emotions and behaviour have become more clear (Dolcos et al.,
2020; Riddell, 2018). For instance, we can safely assert that what we think about,
our emotions and feelings, as well as our behaviours, change both the physical
structure of our brain and the neural functioning of circuits involved (Dolcos et al.,
2020; King, 2019; McEwen, 2007). As a result, we know that optimal functioning
requires the brain to be in a state of adaptivity and executive functioning (Caprara
et al., 2009; Colino, 2022; Lambert et al., 2009; Peters, 2005), which, in turn, requires the activation of the pre-frontal cortex (King, 2019).

In relation to our FOF, then, we know and understand that our coaching language and dialogue can influence a client's functioning through their response to
our questions and how they are engaged during the care process. For example,
researchers Newburg and Waldman (2013) report that words and phrases which
can scarcely be heard influence body and brain changes. The spoken word, our
language, sculpts our sense of self, creating personal and cultural narratives and
discourses (Agarwal, 2020; Bamberg, 2011), as well as pro- and anti-social behaviour, our decision-making, and even our thoughts and feelings (Sapolsky, 2017).
The right side of the FOF offers a framework to guide the coach's language and
questioning asking to facilitate optimal functioning, by linking those dialogic skills
and tools with our understanding of how those choices influence the brain and
body. Although a description of all these skills and tools is beyond the scope of this
chapter, we can provide a story to illustrate how the funnel was used to transform
nursing teams' perceptions and experiences of a new behaviour support program
implemented in our hospital, leading to more optimal functioning of staff across
our in-patient units.

The Funnel in Practice

Almost two years ago, during the receding COVID-19 healthcare crisis, our hospital received funding for a program to support staff mental health. Throughout and
post COVID, staff reported higher than normal volumes of escalated behaviours
from clients and families. On top of a system bursting from constraints, this perceived amplification of challenging/interfering behaviours seemed in some ways
to be the proverbial straw. Staff simply didn't feel they had the individual or collective capacity to deal with something that was making an already untenable situation even worse. Following extensive consultation, leadership committed to an
education and training program designed to help staff better understand these challenging behaviours and to communicate and engage with clients and families in
ways that support more positive behaviour from them. Ultimately, we expected the
education and training would improve the rapport, engagement and relationships
with clients and families, while reducing the likelihood of escalations and thereby
improving the working conditions and mental health of staff.

In the midst of a staffing shortage, leaders and manager worked diligently to
create schedules for nurses and staff on in-patient units, backfilling to cover for
staff who were attending these half-day training sessions. The harder we worked

to make the program work, the more frustrated everyone became. Our facilitators were discouraged by turnout at the education sessions and the apathy of the staff who showed up. We were at a loss. We knew the program could help, we knew staff wanted and needed a solution and that the program might even be transformative, yet despite our best efforts we failed to get the traction everyone needed. Finally, 18 months and a significant financial and emotional investment by our team later, we sat down and began to ask ourselves different questions. Instead of brainstorming ways to better engage staff, better schedule staff and better convince them of the program's value, a team member asked, "Where do we think staff might be on the funnel?" The answer was easy. The bottom. Knowing where they were on the funnel provided the answer to the next question, "So, what's our strategy?" Again, the answer was easy. We hold space. Now we had an understanding of what they really needed and wanted. Using our funnel skills/tools to determine what we needed to do (and not do) to support them, we designed an entirely new approach. We noticed, strategized, and supported.

Immediately, we cancelled all the formal learning sessions because at the bottom of the funnel people cannot process information in ways that are helpful or useful to them, they need their pre-frontal cortex for learning (the top of the funnel). Instead, we decided we would hold space by providing in-situ coaching support for individuals and/or teams who had or were expecting to have what they perceived to be challenging clients. Our trained coaches (four) were (are) on site five days a week, during the work day, to debrief with staff, in ways the staff determine are best for them. Our coaches wear pagers, so staff can reach them on an urgent basis. Staff can even request that a coach be present in the client's room while they provide care (the coaches never engage with clients and families, only staff). Following the care intervention, the coach and staff member(s) have a real-time conversation about what went well and what they might consider doing differently next time. Staff are now supported in a variety of contexts and situations where they may not feel fully comfortable or confident. Their competency is never judged, only facilitated. By holding space, safe spaces for individuals to show up as their best selves have been created and, as a result, staff are beginning to respond in transformational ways.

It took us about six months of holding space for our staff to move up the funnel enough that managers and supervisors are now asking for the formal learning, and ways to expand the support and training to ambulatory clinics. Although it took us far longer than necessary, given this is what we teach, as a team, we learned how valuable the FOF is as a guide to understanding behaviour – whether individual, or teams – and the strategies and tools to create relationships and care that promote and sustain optimal functioning. We literally learned to practise what we teach. Our coaches now round with teams, consult with the BCBAs (board-certified behaviour analysts), provide informal learning opportunities to teams and meet with teams prior to procedures that may involve a behaviour escalation, or where staff may not feel confident. Perhaps most significantly, we now provide one-on-one coaching to all new hires, in an effort to support their optimal functioning as they transition into a new role, a new organization and a new culture.

Summary

Dr Rachel Remen suggests (2014) that by seeing and enabling the inherent wholeness of others, we make it real. As healthcare providers and practitioners, we have to learn to see wholeness instead of brokenness and we must learn to speak to the wholeness present in all people. When we communicate in ways that enable the inherent strengths and resources of clients and that facilitate the basic human desire of self-actualization, we help these individuals to become the authors and authority of their own healthcare journey. A journey where we become privileged collaborators. Through this collaboration, our healthcare systems can be healed.

Keywords: Humanistic Education and Training

What we use	*What it replaces/how used*
Despite	Problem-focused questioning
Instead	Problem-focused questioning
Suppose	Trying to convince client of next steps
For you	A constraint perspective to minimize overwhelm
What else	The inclination to ask another question without fully engaging the client's agency
Who else	Helps to enhance relationships and client perspective
What	Replaces why questions
Manage	Enhances coping
Do-ing	Replaces feeling questions
Difference	Elicits critical thinking and agency
Helpful/useful	Collaborative goal setting, replaces clinicians' expertise as the only source of expertise
Notice	Elicits enduring personal resources
Might	Replaces: should, can, is
Curious	Replaces a directive approach
Even just a little	A constraint that reduces overwhelm
Good enough	Replaces perfectionist tendencies and constrains overwhelm
And	Replaces but

References

Abington, A. (2013). Croydon Health Services NHS Trust creates an internal-coaching culture: New skills promote organizational change and performance. *Human Resource Management International Digest, 21*(4), 6–11.

Agarwal, V. (2020). *Medical Humanism, Chronic Illness, and the Body in Pain: An Ecology of Wholeness*. Lexington Books.

Bamberg, M. (2011). Who am I? Narration and its contribution to self and identity. *Theory & Psychology, 21*(1), 3–24.

Berg, S. (2022). Pandemic pushes U.S. doctor burnout to all time high of 63%. American Medical Association. Available at: https://www.ama-assn.org/practice-management/physician-health/pandemic-pushes-us-doctor-burnout-all-time-high-63

Boehmer, K.R., Barakat, S., Ahn, S., Prokop, L.J., Erwin, P.J., & Murad, M.H. (2016). Health coaching interventions for persons with chronic conditions: A systematic review and meta-analysis protocol. *Systematic Reviews, 5*(1), 1–7.

Brend, Y. (2022). Health care is showing the cracks it's had for decades. Why it will take more than cash to fix it. CBC News. Available at: https://www.cbc.ca/news/canada/health-care-how-we-got-here-fix-broken-cracks-billions-canadian-duclos-1.6691196#:~:text=But%20fissures%20in%20the%20system,Health%20Data%20Strategy%20in%202021

Caprara, G.V., Fagnani, C., Alessandri, G., Steca, P., Gigantesco, A., Sforza, L.L.C., & Stazi, M.A. (2009). Human optimal functioning: The genetics of positive orientation towards self, life, and the future. *Behavior Genetics, 39*(3), 277–284.

Colino, S. (2022). How stress can damage your brain and body. Washington Post, April 26. Available at: https://www.washingtonpost.com/wellness/2022/04/26/inner-workings-stress-how-it-affects-your-brain-body/?utm_source=instagram&utm_medium=social&utm_campaign=wp_main&crl8_id=acf88cd8-e65d-4232-b9f2-990908c573d8

Cook, E. (2022). The funnel of optimal functioning: A model of coach education. *Coaching Psychologist, 18*(2), 42–57.

Diener, E., Pressman, S.D., Hunter, J., & Delgadillo-Chase, D. (2017). If, why, and when subjective well-being influences health, and future needed research. *Applied Psychology: Health and Well-Being, 9*(2), 133–167.

Dolcos, F., Katsumi, Y., Shen, C., Bogdan, P. C., Jun, S., Larsen, R. et al. (2020). The impact of focused attention on emotional experience: A functional MRI investigation. *Cognitive, Affective, & Behavioral Neuroscience, 20*(5), 1011–1026.

Dubé, K., Willard-Grace, R., O'Connell, B., DeVore, D., Prado, C., Bodenheimer, T., & Thom, D.H. (2015). Clinician perspectives on working with health coaches: A mixed methods approach. *Families, Systems, & Health, 33*(3), 213–21.

Dyrbye, L.N., Shanafelt, T.D., Gill, P.R., Satele, D.V., & West, C.P. (2019). Effect of a professional coaching intervention on the well-being and distress of physicians: A pilot randomized clinical trial. *JAMA Internal Medicine, 179*(10), 1406–1414.

Edwards, C. (2023). Why is Britain's health service, a much-loved national treasure, falling apart? CNN. Available at: https://www.cnn.com/2023/01/23/uk/uk-nhs-crisis-falling-apart-gbr-intl/index.html

Green, L.S., Oades, L.G., & Grant, A.M. (2006). Cognitive-behavioral, solution-focused life coaching: Enhancing goal striving, well-being, and hope. *Journal of Positive Psychology, 1*(3), 142–149.

Green, S. & Palmer, S. (2018). Positive psychology coaching: Science into practice. In *Positive Psychology Coaching in Practice* (pp. 1–15). Routledge.

Haus, M. (2017). Partnerships between the patient and the healthcare delivery chain. *Current Allergy & Clinical Immunology, 30*(1), 6–10.

Kibe, C. & Boniwell, I. (2015). Teaching well-being and resilience in primary and secondary school. In: S. Joseph (ed.), *Positive Psychology in Practice: Promoting Human Flourishing in Work, Health, Education, and Everyday Life* (pp. 297–312). Wiley.

King, G., Chiarello, L.A., Ideishi, R., Ziviani, J., Phoenix, M., McLarnon, M.J. et al. (2021). The complexities and synergies of engagement: An ethnographic study of engagement in outpatient pediatric rehabilitation sessions. *Disability and Rehabilitation, 43*(16), 2353–2365.

King, G., Schwellnus, H., Servais, M., & Baldwin, P. (2019). Solution=focused coaching in pediatric rehabilitation: Investigating transformative experiences and outcomes for families. *Physical & Occupational Therapy in Pediatrics, 39*(1), 16–32.

King, M. (2019). The neural correlates of well-being: A systematic review of the human neuroimaging and neuropsychological literature. *The Psychonomic Society, 19*, 779–796.

Kumagai, A., Richardson, L., Khan, S., & Kuper, A. (2018). Dialogues on the threshold: Dialogical learning for humanism and justice. *Academic Medicine, 93*(12), 1778–1784.

Lambert, K., Eisch, A.J., Galea, L.A., Kempermann, G., & Merzenich, M. (2019). Optimizing brain performance: Identifying mechanisms of adaptive neurobiological plasticity. *Neuroscience & Biobehavioral Reviews, 105*(6184), 60–71.

Leng, L. (2022). Commentary: Healthcare workers are at their breaking point but most don't want to quit. Channel New Asia. Available at: https://www.channelnewsasia.com/commentary/frontline-workers-burnout-covid-19-quit-leave-hospital-doctor-nurse-health-2553806

Linley, P., Joseph, S., Harrington, S., & Wood, A. (2006). Positive psychology: Past, present, and (possible) future. *Journal of Positive Psychology, 1*(1), 3–16.

Lyubomirsky, S., Tkach, C., & DiMatteo, M.R. (2006). What are the differences between happiness and self-esteem? *Social Indicators Research, 78*(3), 363–404.

MacLeod, M.L., Stewart, N.J., Kulig, J.C., Anguish, P., Andrews, M.E., Banner, D. et al. (2017). Nurses who work in rural and remote communities in Canada: A national survey. *Human Resources for Health, 15*(1), 1–11.

Maini, A., Fyfe, M., & Kumar, S. (2020). Medical students as health coaches: Adding value for patients and students. *BMC Medical Education, 20*(182), 182.

Manzi, A., Hirschhorn, L.R., Sherr, K., Chirwa, C., Baynes, C., & Awoonor-Williams, J.K. (2017). Mentorship and coaching to support strengthening healthcare systems: Lessons learned across the five population health implementation and training partnership projects in sub-Saharan Africa. *BMC Health Services Research, 17*(3), 5–16.

Marano, G., Traversi, G., Gesualdi, A., Biffi, A., Gaetani, E., Sani, G., & Mazza, M. (2021). Mental health and coaching challenges facing the COVID-19 outbreak. *Psychiatria Danubina, 33*(1), 124–126.

McEvoy, J. & Thompson, S. (2022). Healthcare burnout in Canada: Facing the problem and creating solutions to better support healthcare works. The National. Available at: https://www.national.ca/en/perspectives/detail/healthcare-burnout/

McEwen, B.S. (2007). Physiology and neurobiology of stress and adaptation: Central role of the brain. *Physiological Reviews, 87*(3), 873–904.

Nafstad, H.E. (2015). Historical, philosophical and epistemological perspectives. In: S. Joseph (ed.), *Positive Psychology in Practice: Promoting Human Flourishing in Work, Health, Education, and Everyday Life* (pp. 9–30). Wiley.

Newburg, A. & Waldman, M. (2013). *Words Can Change Your Brain: 12 Conversational Strategies to Build Trust, Resolve Conflict and Increase Intimacy*. Penguin Books.

Peters, E. (2005). *Neuropsychological Executive Functioning and Psychosocial Well-Being*. Doctoral dissertation, North-West University.

Reinhart, E. (2023). Doctors aren't burned out from overwork. We're demoralized by our health system. New York Times. Available at: https://www.nytimes.com/2023/02/05/opinion/doctors-universal-health-care.html

Reis, T., Faria, I., Serra, H., & Xavier, M. (2022). Barriers and facilitators to implementing a continuing medical education intervention in a primary health care setting. *BMC Health Services Research, 22*(1), 638.

Remen, R. (1999). Helping, fixing or serving? Mental Health Association of San Francisco. Available at: https://www.mentalhealthsf.org/wp-content/uploads/2020/01/HelpingFixingServing-by-Rachel-Remen.pdf

Remen, R. (2014). Becoming a blessing. Youtube, uploaded by Bioneers, December 22. Available at: https://www.youtube.com/watch?v=77tM-gEzA14

Riddell, P. (2018). Coaching and neuroscience. In: S. Palmer & A. Whybrow (eds), *Handbook of Coaching Psychology* (pp. 14–24). Routledge.

Rider, E., Gilligan, M., Osterberg, L., Litzelman, D., Plews-Ogan, M., Weil, A. et al. (2018). Healthcare at the Crossroads: The need to shape an organizational culture of humanistic teaching and practice. *Journal of General Internal Medicine, 33*(7), 1092–1099.

Rogers, C.R. (1979). The foundations of the person-centered approach. *Education, 100*(2), 98–107.

Palamara, K., Kauffman, C., Stone, V.E., Bazari, H., & Donelan, K. (2015). Promoting success: A professional development coaching program for interns in medicine. *Journal of Graduate Medical Education, 7*(4), 630–637.

Sapolsky, R. (2017). *Behave: The Biology of Humans at Our Best and Worst*. Penguin Books.

Schneider, K.J., Bugental, J.F.T., & Pierson, J.F. (2001). Closing statements. In: *The Handbook of Humanistic Psychology* (pp. 667–675). SAGE Publications.

Schwellnus, H., King, G., & Thompson, L. (2015). Client-centred coaching in the paediatric health professions: A critical scoping review. *Disability and Rehabilitation, 37*(15), 1305–1315.

Seko, Y., King, G., Keenan, S., Maxwell, J., Oh, A., & Curran, C.J. (2020). Impact of solution-focused coaching training on pediatric rehabilitation specialists: A longitudinal evaluation study. *Journal of Interprofessional Care, 34*(4), 481–492.

Surr, C.A., Parveen, S., Smith, S.J., Drury, M., Sass, C., Burden, S., & Oyebode, J. (2020). The barriers and facilitators to implementing dementia education and training in health and social care services: A mixed-methods study. *BMC Health Services Research, 20*, 1–10.

van den Goor, M. Boerebach, B., Bindels, E., Heineman, M.J., & Lombarts, K. (2020). The doctor's heart: A qualitative study exploring physicians' views on their professional performance in light of excellence, humanistic practice and accountability. *Research Square.* DOI: https://doi.org/10.21203/re.3.rs-22857/v1

van Nieuwerburgh, C. & Oades, L. (2017). Editorial. Coaching: An International Journal of Theory, Research & Practice, *11*(2), 99–101.

Warby, T. (2022). Why Australia needs a systemic response to burnout. Royal Australian College of General Practitioners. Available at: https://www1.racgp.org.au/newsgp/gp-opinion/why-australia-needs-a-systemic-response-to-burnout

Wolff, M., Hammoud, M., Santen, S., Deiorio, N., & Fix, M. (2020). Coaching in undergraduate medical education: A national survey. *Medical Education Online, 25*(1), article 1699765.

World Health Organization (WHO). (2023). The health workforce crisis in Europe is no longer a looming threat – it is here and now. The Bucharest Declaration charts a way forward. Available at: https://www.who.int/europe/news/item/22-03-2023-the-health-workforce-crisis-in-europe-is-no-longer-a-looming-threat—it-is-here-and-now-the-bucharest-declaration-charts-a-way-forward

Zulman, D.M., Haverfield, M.C., Shaw, J.G., Brown-Johnson, C.G., Schwartz, R., Tierney, A. et al. (2020). Practices to foster physician presence and connection with patients in the clinical encounter. *JAMA, 323*(1), 70–81.

2 A Humanistic, Solution-Focused Approach to Person-Centred Care and Client-Activation

Gilbert J. Greene

A basic tenet in healthcare today is that it should be evidence-based. This position first entered professional literature in 1990 and is commonly referred to as evidence-based medicine (EBM, Eddy, 2011). EBM involves making treatment decisions based on the best scientific information available which is found in randomized controlled trials, peer-reviewed studies, systematic reviews, and meta-analyses (Siegel et al., 2023, p. 903). The common understanding of EBM is that it involves technical aspects of bio-medical care such as specific medical interventions, surgical procedures, techniques, medications, and so on. Traditional EBM practice is *clinician-centred* in that the healthcare provider (HCP) is the expert, with the emphasis on their professional and technical knowledge and expertise, and the client is a passive recipient of such knowledge and expertise. However, treatment is not going to be effective without the client's (patient's) *buy-in* to the treatment regimen and engaging in self-care (Sullivan, 2017).

In recent years, some have advocated for expanding EBM to evidence-based practice (EBP), which includes all of EBM, as well as learning and using the client's (patient's) values and preferences in developing and maintaining a collaborative relationship with the client and getting their buy-in to treatment (Siegel et al., 2023). In treatment, the evidence-based technical knowledge and clinical expertise do come unilaterally from the clinician, thus making it *clinician-centred*. But a clinician-centred approach can encourage and reinforce clients' responding passively to the treatment regimen and not buying into it; that is, not actively engaging in self-management and doing their part in achieving positive outcomes. How, then, does the clinician learn and use the client's values, preferences, and perspectives in getting client (patient) buy-in and successfully implementing EBP in their lives? This chapter aims to discuss how to effectively operationalize this using a humanistic, solution-focused approach.

Person-Centred Care

For starters, you may have noticed that I have already used the term "client" instead of "patient." We use the term "client" instead of "patient" given that the latter is associated with the more narrow, hierarchical clinician-centred bio-medical approach of EBM and connotes "passivity."

DOI: 10.4324/9781003414490-3

In recent years, three approaches have grown in popularity for effectively learn-ing how to develop and maintain a collaborative relationship with clients, espe-cially by using their values, preferences, goals, and perspectives in ways that create a context for clients to take a more active role in their healthcare: *patient-centered healthcare* (Fortin VI et al., 2019), *person-centered healthcare* (McCormack et al., 2021), and *relationship-centred healthcare* (Chou & Cooley, 2018). Although these three approaches have some different emphases, often the terms are used inter-changeably (Flieger, 2017).

There is a considerable amount of literature on all three of these perspectives and, overall, there is little difference between the three (Beach et al., 2006; Fridberg et al., 2022; Grover et al., 2022; Rider, 2011; The American Geriatrics Society Expert Panel on Person-Centered Care, 2015). In addition, studies have found all three perspectives to be effective on the same outcomes such as client satisfaction with care, and cost-effectiveness (Capko & Bisera, 2014; Chou & Cooley, 2018; McCormack et al., 2021). Thus, it can be said that developing and maintaining col-laborative relationships with clients is an EBP.

Clinicians developing and maintaining a collaborative relationship with clients is the foundation of all three approaches. Most of the skills necessary for devel-oping such a relationship are based on the work of humanistic psychologist Carl Rogers, who developed *client-centred therapy* which he later called *person-centred therapy* (1965, 1978). Because of the common use of the skills of person-centred therapy, throughout the rest of this chapter, I will use the term *person-centred care (PCC)* or *person-centred approaches (PCAs)* to refer to all three approaches. Below are the common features of the person-centred approaches:

- Take a humanistic approach in providing care.
  - View the person as whole and engage in holistic healthcare.
- Elicit client's narrative.
- Establish and maintain a positive clinician–client relationship.
  - Empathy
  - Unconditional positive regard (warmth)
  - Genuineness (authenticity)
- Support client self-determination, autonomy, and empowerment by privileging clients' preferences, values, and goals.
- Develop and maintain a collaborative relationship with the client and all in-volved in the client's care, such as family members and other providers of care.
- Support client activation (choices, strengths, competencies, resources).

Carl Rogers' Person-Centred Approach

At the heart of PCAs is how the clinician communicates with the client. It is impor-tant for the clinician to communicate with the client in a way that elicits the client's narrative about their concerns, values, and preferences. For this to occur, clients

need to feel safe with and be able to trust the clinician. How the clinician responds
to the client's narrative is the vehicle for initially developing such a relationship
and the person-centred approach that Carl Rogers developed has been found to be
a very effective way for doing this.

A fundamental belief of Carl Rogers' person-centred approach is the "actualizing tendency" of all living organisms, including humans (Rogers, 1963). According to the actualizing tendency, all organisms move in the direction of maintaining
and enhancing themselves. In regard to this, Rogers states "… it is my belief that
there is one central source of energy in the human organism; that it is a function
of the whole organism rather than of some portion of it; and that it is perhaps best
conceptualized as a tendency toward fulfillment, toward actualization, toward the
maintenance and enhancement of the organism" (1963, p. 6). Thus, in therapy, the
client is seen as having the inherent capacity to change; or as Bohart, a person-
centred therapist, states, the client becomes a "self-healer" (Bohart, 2000).

The actualizing tendency is always operating, but is especially effective when
conditions are optimal. For Carl Rogers (1957), the optimal conditions for humans
occur in a relational context in which the other person responds with empathy, unconditional positive regard (warmth/accepting), and genuineness (congruence). In
therapy, these are three core conditions the clinician must provide to the client to
create a context for change. At the same time, it is necessary for the client to perceive and experience the clinician as providing these conditions. Rogers claimed
that providing these conditions was not only necessary, but also sufficient for therapy to be successful. However, subsequent research over the years has found that
the clinician needs to do more than Rogers suggests (Watson, 2007).

Therapeutic Alliance

Person-centred therapy is one of many different *bona fide* approaches to psychotherapy. Meta-analyses of psychotherapy outcome studies conducted over many
years have found that all *bona fide* therapeutic approaches are effective and no one
approach is more effective than any other. *Bona fide* therapies are defined as "those
that are delivered by trained therapists and are based on psychological principles,
are offered to the psychotherapy community as viable treatments (e.g., through professional books or manuals), or contained specified components" (Wampold et al.,
1997, p. 205). What accounts for therapeutic success are factors they all have in
common (Wampold, 2019; Wampold & Imel, 2015). The most potent of these factors is the alliance between the clinician and client; this has been found to be true
for psychotherapy (Wampold & Fluckiger, 2023) and coaching (Grabman et al.,
2020). The therapeutic alliance has been operationalized as consisting of *positive
affective bonds* between the clinician and client (which would be developed and
maintained using Rogers' core conditions), *mutual agreement on goals* for treatment, and *mutual agreement on tasks* for achieving the goals. These last elements of
the therapeutic alliance were not explicit parts of Rogers' person-centred approach.

Another important factor in therapy being successful is the client's "buy-in" to
the treatment the clinician is offering. For clients to buy into the treatment, they

must have a positive relationship with the clinician, that is, they must feel safe and trust the clinician and feel the clinician understands and cares about them as a person. In addition, the treatment needs to fit the client's values, beliefs, and frames of reference. A central emphasis of PCAs is clinicians developing a clinician–client relationship whereby the client buys into and becomes an *active participant* in their healthcare and maintenance. Meta-analyses have found these factors to hold true in both behavioural and bio-medical healthcare (Wampold & Fluckiger, 2023).

Patient Activation

Clients' self-management is important to their well-being and treatment outcomes. For clients to engage in behaviours consistent with self-management, it is important for them to believe they can accomplish their health goals. In other words, they need to have a sense of *personal agency* (Little et al., 2006). Personal agency is on a continuum with those low in personal agency lacking confidence that they can accomplish certain goals and thus being passive and not taking necessary action; whereas those high on personal agency are confident they can achieve their goals regardless of the challenges they might encounter. Constructs related to personal agency are self-efficacy, locus of control, and empowerment.

A challenge in healthcare is clients who are passive about taking care of their health and well-being and not following through on the preferred treatments and lifestyle. A clinician can be the best trained, qualified, and technically skilled, but clients not actively participating in their healthcare can limit treatment effectiveness and be financially costly. This process is referred to as *patient activation* (PA; Hibbard et al., 2005). Patient activation involves an individual's knowledge, skill, and confidence for managing their health, healthcare, and disease (Hibbard et al., 2004). Like personal agency, PA is on a continuum.

To measure patient activation, Hibbard et al. (2004, 2005) developed the Patient Activation Measure (PAM) for physical health and Green et al. (2010) developed one for mental health. The PAM consists of 13 items and is scored on a 4-point Likert scale: disagree strongly, disagree, agree, and agree strongly with a not applicable option. Numerous studies on patient activation as measured by the PAM have been conducted in different settings, for different clinical problems, and in a variety of countries. Below are the items of the PAM for bio-medical settings:

1　When all is said and done, I am the person who is responsible for managing my health condition.
2　Taking an active role in my own healthcare is the most important factor in determining my health and ability to function.
3　I am confident that I can take actions that will help prevent or minimize some symptoms or problems associated with my health condition.
4　I know what each of my prescribed medications do.
5　I am confident that I can tell when I need to go get medical care and when I can handle a health problem myself.

6   I am confident I can tell my healthcare provider concerns I have even when he or she does not ask.
7   I am confident that I can follow through on medical treatments I need to do at home.
8   I understand the nature and causes of my health condition(s).
9   I know the different medical treatment options available for my health condition.
10 I have been able to maintain the lifestyle change for my health that I have made.
11 I know how to prevent further problems with my health condition.
12 I am confident that I can figure out solutions when new situations or problems arise with my health condition.
13 I am confident that I can maintain lifestyle changes like diet and exercise even during times of stress.

Studies have found that clients with low PA can experience increases in their activation levels through certain clinician behaviours such as those consistent with the PCAs listed above. Despite the effectiveness of the PCAs for improving PA, there has been little discussion on how to specifically operationalize certain processes such as collaboration, goal setting, and working with client resources (strengths and competencies). This latter clinician activity has been referred to as *resource activation*.

Resource Activation

Frequently, at the very beginning of treatment, clients say they are stuck. They have tried everything they know to do, and nothing has worked. Others they may have consulted, such as friends, family, or other professional helpers, have not been helpful either. The client and these other helpers have focused on "fixing the problem" and remediating the client's deficits. Consequently, the client at this point is usually feeling inadequate, discouraged, and hopeless, resulting in taking a passive stance towards trying to change and making things better (Fluckiger et al., 2009). What they and their helpers have not appreciated is that people are more than their problems and deficits; they also have *strengths* and *competencies* that are going unused or underused. However, their strengths and competencies are *resources* that can be activated in the service of them achieving their goals and making the changes they want (Fluckiger et al., 2010; Grawe, 1997). The clinician activating clients' resources is the "motor that drives the therapeutic endeavor ... the alpha and omega of effective therapy" (Grawe, 1997, p. 6). But how do clinicians and clients working together do this?

I mentioned above that numerous studies and meta-analyses have found that no one theoretical approach to therapy is more effective than any other. However, there is growing evidence that therapy in which the clinician and client talk more about the client's resources, especially in how they can be used to achieve the clients' goals, the better the outcomes. That is, *resource-activated therapy* is more effective than non-resource-activated therapy (Fluckiger et al., 2023; Munder et al., 2019; Schurmann-Vengels et al., 2022).

In the beginning of the development of RA, the approach to activating client resources was rather general (Fluckiger & Holtforth, 2008). Clients were initially assessed, including for their strengths. Before each session for the first five sessions, a trained master's student met with the therapist for 5 minutes to discuss the client's strengths and how the therapist might activate resources with the client in the coming session; this was referred to as a "priming intervention." After the session, the graduate student met with the therapist again for 5 minutes to review how the therapist did resource activation during the session. However, not long after the initial development of RA, its creators began discussing using *solution-focused therapy* and interventions unique to it to activate client resources.

The Solution-Focused Approach

The solution-focused approach (SFA) believes that people are much more than their problems and deficits and posits that the quickest way to help a person achieve positive change is by identifying and amplifying their resources (strengths, competencies, and skills). The SFA takes a non-normative and non-pathological view and thus is not interested in labels or diagnosis and does not try to rectify deficits or fix or heal pathology. In this way, the SFA is humanistic.

Although the SFA originated in a setting for providing psychotherapy, it has evolved to be a way of thinking and communicating in general.

An underpinning of the SFA is social constructionism; that is, one's perception of reality is socially co-constructed through conversation/dialogue with others. Thus, what we talk about we create and reinforce. If we focus on discussing with a person their problems, deficits, and negative emotions, they end up feeling more negatively, pessimistic, and demoralized; whereas if we focus on talking with them about their strengths, competencies, and skills, they end up feeling more positive emotions, optimistic, and hopeful (Greene & Lee, 2011). Meta-analyses have found the solution-focused approach to be efficacious in a variety of settings with various presenting problems (Franklin et al., 2023; Karababa, 2024; Kim et al., 2019; Zhang et al., 2018). Several assumptions and guidelines have evolved that help to operationalize the SFA with some consistency.

Assumptions and Guidelines

All people have strengths, competencies, and resources. This is a fundamental belief of the SFA. The job of the clinician is, through dialogue with the client, to find and activate that part of the client that knows how not to have the problem or how to have less of the problem.

Change is happening all the time. Even when someone has a chronic problem, there are times when it is less frequent or intense. Rather than ask about when the problem is at its worst, we want to find out when is the problem better and what is different at those times? What does the client do to get those better times to happen?

Engage in solution and change talk rather than problem and deficit talk. As mentioned above, what we talk about we create. There will be times when the client will want to talk about the problem. When the clinician and client first meet, the initial conversation will usually be about the problem. When the clinician feels it appropriate, he or she should bring the conversation back to talking about solutions, resources, and change.

Focus on the present and future rather than the past. Usually, when the client starts off talking about the problem, he or she will also talk about the past when the problem began and the history of the problem. It is through how the clinician responds to the client when the client talks about the problem and the past that a positive therapeutic relationship is developed. However, the clinician does not want to spend any more time than necessary engaging with the client in talking about the problem and the past.

Small change can lead to larger change. All behaviour is contextual (interpersonal and physical environment). Individuals respond to their contexts and through their interactions individuals and their contexts mutually influence each other. Thus, a change in one part of the context can affect other parts of the context and it can take only a small change to create a "ripple effect" leading to larger change.

Clients are the experts. Clinicians need to have expertise in knowing how to structure a conversation and meeting with the client that will be productive. However, because reality is socially constructed, clients are experts on their reality and lives. Consequently, clinicians *lead from one step behind.*

If it doesn't work do something different; if it does work do more of it. The clinician wants to find out what the client sees as the problem and what the client has done to try to solve the problem. By finding out what has not worked thus far, the client and the clinician discover what not to do. And when there are times when the problem is not present, the client can do more of what they did at those times.

It is much easier to change what we do than who we are. Clinicians should use open-ended follow-up questions to get clients to provide very behaviourally specific descriptions of problems, goals, solutions, etc., commonly asking something like "What will you be doing instead?" or "What will that look like?"

Use pre-suppositional questions. Instead of asking something like "if you change?" instead ask "when you change?" Worded this way, the question pre-supposes the client's desired change will occur.

Solution-Focused Conversational Tools

Because one's definition of reality (beliefs/taken-for-granted assumptions) is socially constructed in dialogue, language use is very important in the SFA (Greene & Lee, 2002; Greene et al., 2005). To further operationalize the SFA, clinicians use several questions unique to it for identifying, activating, and amplifying client resources and solutions, thus leading to clients achieving their self-determined goals.

Exception questions. Because change is happening all the time, there are times when the problem is not present or at least is a little bit better. In the SFA, the emphasis is on the clinician asking the client to identify those times. Once the client identifies an exception, it is important for the clinician to follow up and ask questions to obtain a detailed description of those times. With exception questions, we are asking about *current or recent exceptions*. For example:

- "When are there times you do exercise, even just a little bit?"
- "What's different at those times?"

For a problem that may involve impulsivity or compulsivity, the clinician might ask something like:

- "When are there times you feel like having a drink, but you don't? How are you able to do that?"

Questions for identifying past exceptions. Sometimes the client cannot identify a current or recent exception, so we ask for past exceptions regardless of how long ago that occurred.

Miracle question. As mentioned previously, the SFA emphasizes talking about the future more than the past. One way to invite the client into talking about the future is asking the miracle question. Asking the miracle question is a way to have the client define their desired outcome goals, but it is also an intervention in itself. To answer the question, the client has to create an image of what will be different after the miracle. Consequently, the miracle question invites the client into a process of "unguided imagery."

Clinician: Let me ask you a strange question.
Client: Ok.
Clinician: Suppose that after our meeting you go home and then this evening you go to bed for the night (pause) and while you are sleeping tonight, (pause) a miracle happens and the miracle is the problem you came to see me about is suddenly solved; like magic the problem is gone (pause). However, because you were sleeping, you don't know that a miracle happened, (pause) but when you wake up tomorrow morning, you will be different (pause). So when you first wake up in the morning, how will you know a miracle has happened? (pause) What will be the *first small sign* that you will notice when you first wake up that will indicate to you that the problem is solved?

After the client responds, then the clinician needs to ask follow-up questions to get detailed behavioural indicators of the "miracle picture;" doing so makes it more real and doable.

- "What difference will that make to you?"
- "Who will be the first to notice?"
- "What will he or she notice different about you?"
- "How will they respond differently to you?"

- "How will you respond to them?"
- "What difference will that make?"
- "Who will be the first to notice at school/work?"
- "What will they notice different about you?"
- "How will they respond to you?"
- "How will you respond to them?"
- "Is that different?"
- "What difference will that make?"
- "How might the rest of your day go?"

Notice the pauses in the miracle question above. How the clinician asks the miracle question is very important to its effectiveness. You want to ask the question slowly and with a soft tone of voice. The pausing helps slow down the process and allows for the clinician to see if the question is resonating with the client.

Scaling questions. A lot of clients think and talk in broad generalities and in either/or binary terms; doing this can limit possibilities and options. In using the scaling question, the clinician can ask the client to scale anything that may seem important and relevant, such as feelings or level of motivation. The scaling question can be especially helpful in assessing and monitoring progress.

The SFA uses a 10–0 scale where 10 is the best and 0 is the worst. For example, a clinician could ask a client how hopeful they are about the future; here, 10 represents feeling completely hopeful and 0 no hope at all. The 10–0 scale shown below can be used to ask the client to rank the primary presenting concern at the first session and then every session afterwards to monitor progress.

In using the scaling question for ranking the problem and goal, the clinician will ask the client to rank the problem and their desired outcome goal on the 10–0 scale, where 10 is the complete absence of the problem and achievement of the goal and 0 is the worst the problem could be. The clinician can graphically represent the scale continuum like the following:

Complete achievement of the goal   The worst the problem could be
(complete absence of the problem)

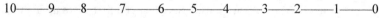

10———9———8———7———6———5———4———3———2———1———0

- First, ask the client to define their desired outcome goal as concretely and specifically as possible with as many behavioural indicators as possible in terms of who, what, when, where, how, and how often (use the client's description/ definition), and then have the client rank the problem on the 10–0 scale.
- Next, ask the client to define their presenting problem as concretely and specifically as possible with as many behavioural indicators as possible in terms of who, what, when, where, how, and how often (use the client's description/ definition), and then have the client rank the problem on the 10–0 scale.
- Then, ask the client how they will know when they have moved up 1 point from where they currently are on the 10–0 scale – what will that look like and how will other people know when they have moved up 1 point on the scale?

Coping questions. Sometimes clients are not able to identify any exceptions and are constantly feeling overwhelmed. Many find themselves in situations that most anyone would experience as realistically overwhelming, but somehow, the clients keep going every day. An example of a coping question could be:

Clinician: You've been feeling stressed, overwhelmed, and depressed for a long time. How do you cope with your situation? How do you keep going every day?

Client: I do it for my kids. I have to get up and keep going. There's no one else to take care of them and I really do love them.

A version of the coping question is asking the client "What are you doing to keep the problem from getting worse" when the client reports making no progress on the 10–0 scale.

Personal agency questions. Asking this question is very important to activating and reinforcing the client's sense of agency and empowerment. Several examples have already been demonstrated above. For example, once a client has identified an exception to the problem, the clinician asks, "How did you do that?" or "How do you keep going every day?" etc.

Relationship questions. This is another important follow-up question to the client identifying an exception or answering the miracle question. This question helps to contextualize the desired change. In addition, it invites clients to take the perspective of other people. For example, see the follow-up questions to the miracle question above.

The Solution-Focused Process

1. Engage clients in developing and maintaining a collaborative relationship.

Elicit from and give clients the space to tell their story (narrative). It is how the clinician responds to the client during this telling of the story that the relationship is built and maintained. Right from the beginning of the encounter with the client and throughout the meeting and every meeting thereafter, the clinician should respond with respect, empathy, unconditional positive regard (warmth/acceptance), and genuineness (congruence), validating the client as they tell their story. It is from the clinician's responses such as these that the *positive affective bonds* of the *therapeutic alliance* are developed and maintained.

Also, during this first phase and throughout working with the client, use the *language of collaboration* (Greene & Lee, 2011). In the solution-focused practice world today, it is common to start off meetings with clients with the *best hopes question*, namely, "What are your best hopes for our work together?" or "What are your best hopes for this meeting today?" Examples of other related questions are:

- "How do you want to spend our time together today?"
- "What are you wanting for yourself today?"
- "What concerns of yours do you want to address today?"

- "What can we work on together to achieve what you want for yourself?"
- "How will you know that coming here today was worthwhile?"

2. Define the problem from the client's perspective.

In the SFA, we are more concerned about the client's future and resources, but clients often expect and want to tell their story. They want the clinician to know who they are as a person. Their story includes their problems and concerns. Thus, the clinician should be *genuinely curious* about their story by asking the who, what, where, when, how, and how often questions regarding their story, especially about their concerns and problems.

3. Goal setting.

Working together with clients on their self-determined goals is the essence of collaboration. Getting a well-defined goal is necessary for collaborative work to be focused on the future rather than the past. Clients are much more motivated to work on goals they define for themselves rather than those others define for them (Tryon et al., 2019). For a goal to be well-defined, it should be as follows:

- Important to clients.
- Small and achievable.
- Specific and behavioural – obtain as many behavioural indicators as possible of progress towards and achievement of the goal. Initially, many clients define their problem and goal in very general terms. For example:

Client: I just want to be happy.
Clinician: When you become happy, what will that look like? How will people close to you know that you are happy?

- Seek the presence rather than the absence of something. That is, have clients state the goals in the positive rather than the negative. Frequently, clients define their goal as the absence of the problem. For example:

Client: I want to stop feeling depressed.
Clinician: When you stop feeling depressed, what will you be feeling and doing instead?

The miracle question can be used to get clients to define their goal. Most, but not all, clients respond well to the miracle question. Instead of the miracle question, a clinician can use the 10–0 scale. In addition, you can simply use an *outcome question* such as, "How will you know when you feel that our work together has been successful, and it is time to terminate? What will that look like?"

4. Identifying and amplifying solution patterns (what's happening when things are better/when the problem is less frequent or intense or nonexistent?).

Here, we use all the questions briefly described above. In the SFA, the questions are interventions. They shift the conversation from problem/deficit talk to strength/solution talk; from talking about the past to talking about the future. For example, the client identifies an exception to the problem and then the clinician asks follow-up questions to get details of the exception time. Doing this activates and amplifies the resources the client used to get that exception to happen.

5. Use between-session solution-focused tasks.

Many, but not all, solution-focused clinicians like for clients to do activities between sessions. These activities are in the form of tasks consistent with the client's responses during the meeting. These tasks are suggested at the end of a session right before it ends. There are two general types of between-session tasks: *observational* and *behavioural*. Examples of an observational task are the following:

"Between now and the next time we meet":

• "Pay attention and notice those times you wanted to get off your diet, but you don't. Notice what you did to not give in to the temptation."
• "Pay attention and notice when you have moved up one point on the 10–0 scale. Notice what's different and what you did to get that to happen."

Examples of a behavioral task are the following:

• "For the first hour of every morning, pretend the miracle has happened."
• "You've identified several exceptions to the problem when things are better; so just keep doing what works."

A helpful guide in deciding which type of task to use is the *Funnel of Optimal Functioning* (FOF; Cook, 2022; see also Chapter 1 of this book). If a client is at the lowest end of the FOF, the clinician might not suggest a task, but just compliment the client for coming and participating and for the strengths noted during the meeting. At the middle level of the funnel, the clinician might suggest an observational task and at the highest level a behavioural task.

Conclusion

Evidence-based treatment is not effective if clients are not actively involved in self-management of their physical and mental healthcare. Clients are more than their problems and deficits; they have resources that can be activated in the service of their health. The clinician developing and maintaining a collaborative relationship with the client is critical. To do this, it is important for clinicians to privilege the client's preferences, values, and goals. Identifying and amplifying the client's resources has been found to be a very effective way of doing this.

References

Beach, M.C., Inui, T., & The Relationship-Centered Care Research Network. (2006). Relationship-centered care: A constructive reframing. *Journal of General Internal Medicine, 21*(Suppl. 1), S3–S8.

Bohart, A.C. (2000). The client is the most common factor: Clients' self-healing capacities and psychotherapy. *Journal of Psychotherapy Integration, 10*(2), 127–149.

Capko, J. & Bisera, C. (2014). *The Patient-Centered Payoff: Driving Practice Growth through Image, Culture, and Patient Experience*. Greenbranch Publishing, LLC.

Chou, C. & Cooley, L. (2018). *Communication Rx: Transforming Healthcare through Relationship-Centered Communication*. McGraw Hill.

Cook, E. (2022). The funnel of optimal functioning: A model coach education. *The Coaching Psychologist, 18*(2), 42–57.

Eddy, D.M. (2011). The origins of evidence-based medicine-a personal perspective. *Virtual Mentor, 13*(1), 55–60.

Flieger, S.P. (2017). Implementing the patient-centered medical home in complex adaptive systems: Becoming a relationship-centered patient-centered medical home. *Health Care Management Review, 42*(2), 112–121.

Fluckiger, C., Caspar, F., Holtforth, M.G., & Willutzki, U. (2009). Working with patients' strengths: A microprocess approach. *Psychotherapy Research, 19*(2), 213–223.

Fluckiger, C. & Holtforth, M.G. (2008). Focusing the therapist's attention on the patient's strengths: A preliminary study to foster a mechanism of change in outpatient psychotherapy. *Journal of Clinical Psychology, 64*(7), 876–890.

Fluckiger, C., Munder, T., Del Re, A.C., & Solomonov, N. (2023). Strengths-based methods – a narrative review and comparative multilevel meta-analysis of positive interventions in clinical settings. *Psychotherapy Research, 33*(7), 856–872.

Fluckiger, C., Wusten, G., Zinbarg, R.E., & Wampold, B.E. (2010). *Resource Activation: Using Client's Own Strengths in Psychotherapy and Counseling*. Hogrefe Publishing.

Fortin VI, A.H., Dwamena, F.C., Frankel, R.M., Lepisto, B.L., & Smith, R.C. (2019). *Smith's Patient-Centered Interviewing: An Evidence-Based Method* (4th ed.). McGraw Hill.

Franklin, C., Ding, X., Kim, J., Zhang, A., Hai, A.H., Jones, K. et al. (2023). Solution-focused brief therapy in community-based services: A meta-analysis of randomized controlled studies. *Research on Social Work Practice, 34*(3), 265–276.

Fridberg, H., Wallin, L., & Tistad, M. (2022). Operationalisation of person-centered care in a real-world setting: A case study with six embedded units. *BMC Health Services Research, 22*(1), 1160.

Grabmann, C., Scholmerich, F., & Schermuly, C.C. (2020). The relationship between working alliance and client outcomes in coaching: A meta-analysis. *Human Relations, 73*(2), 35–58.

Grawe, K. (1997). Research-informed psychotherapy. *Psychotherapy Research, 7*(1), 1–19.

Green, C.A., Perrin, N.A., Polen, M.R., Leo, M.C., Hibbard, J.H., & Tusler, M. (2010). Development of the Patient Activation Measure for mental health. *Administration & Policy in Mental Health, 37*(4), 327–333.

Greene, G.J. & Lee, M.Y. (2002). The social construction of empowerment. In: M. O'Melia & K.K. Milley (eds), *Pathways to Power: Readings in Contextual Social Work Practice* (pp. 175–201). Allyn & Bacon.

Greene, G.J. & Lee, M.Y. (2011). *Solution-Oriented Social Work Practice: An Integrative Approach to Working with Client Strengths*. Oxford University Press.

Greene, G.J., Lee, M.Y., & Hoffpauir, S. (2005). The languages of empowerment and strengths in clinical social work: A constructivist perspective. *Families in Society, 86*(2), 267–277.

Grover, S., Fitzpatrick, A., Azim, F.T., Ariza-Vega, P., Bellwood, P., Burns, J. et al. (2022). Defining and implementing patient-centered care: An umbrella review. *Patient Education and Counseling, 105*(7), 1679–1688.

Hibbard, J.H., Mahoney, E.R., Stockard, J., & Tusler, M. (2004). Development of the Patient Activation Measure (PAM): Conceptualizing and measuring activation in patients and consumers. *Health Services Research, 39*(4 Pt 1), 1005–1026.

Hibbard, J.H., Mahoney, E.R., Stockard, J., & Tusler, M. (2005). Development and testing of a short form of the Patient Activation Measure. *Health Services Research, 40*(6 Pt 1), 1918–1930.

Karababa, A. (2024). A meta-analysis of solution-focused brief therapy for school-related problems in adolescents. *Research on Social Work Practice, 34*(51), 169–181.

Kim, J., Jordan, S.S., Franklin, C., & Froerer, A. (2019). Is solution-focused brief therapy evidence-based? An update 10 years later. *Families in Society, 100*(2), 127–138.

Little, T.D., Snyder, C.R., & Wehmeyer, M. (2006). The agentic self: On the nature and origins of personal agency across the life span. In: D.K. Mroczek (ed.), *Handbook of Personality Development* (pp. 61–79). Lawrence Erlbaum Associates Publishers.

McCormack, B., McCance, T., Bulley, C., Brown, D., McMillan, A., & Martin, S. (eds). (2021). *Fundamentals of Person-Centred Healthcare Practice.* John Wiley & Sons, Inc.

Munder, T., Karcher, A., Yadikar, O., Szeles, T., & Gumz, A. (2019). Focusing on patients' existing resources and strengths in cognitive-behavioral therapy and psychodynamic therapy: A systematic review and meta-analysis. *Zeitschrift für Psychosomatische Medizin und Psychotherapie, 65*(2), 144–161.

Rider, E.A. (2011). Advanced communication strategies for relationship-centered care. *Pediatric Annals, 40*(9), 447–453.

Rogers, C.R. (1957). The necessary and sufficient conditions of therapeutic personality change. *Journal of Consulting Psychology, 21*(2), 95–103.

Rogers, C.R. (1963). The actualizing tendency in relation to "motives" and to consciousness. In: M. R. Jones (ed.), *Nebraska Symposium on Motivation,* Vol. XI (pp. 1–24). University of Nebraska Press.

Rogers, C.R. (1965). *Client-Centered Therapy.* Houghton Mifflin.

Rogers, C.R. (1978). *Carl Rogers on Personal Power: Inner Strength and Its Revolutionary Impact.* Trans-Atlantic Publications.

Schurmann-Vengels, J., Teismann, T., Margraf, J., & Willutzki, U. (2022). Patients' self-perceived strengths increase during treatment and predict outcome in outpatient cognitive behavioral therapy. *Journal of Clinical Psychology, 78*(12), 2427–2445.

Siegel, M.G., Lubowitz, J.H., Brand, J.C., & Rossi, M.J. (2023). Evidence-based practice should supersede evidence-based medicine through consideration of clinical experience and patient characteristics in addition to the published literature. *Arthroscopy: The Journal of Arthroscopic and Related Surgery, 39*(4), 903–907.

Sullivan, M.D. (2017). *The Patient as Agent of Health and Health Care.* Oxford University Press.

The American Geriatrics Society Expert Panel on Person-Centered Care. (2015). Person-centered care: A definition and essential elements. *Journal of the American Geriatrics Society, 64*(1), 15–18.

Tryon, G.S., Birch, S.E., & Verkuilen, J. (2019). Goal consensus and collaboration. In: J. C. Norcross & M. J. Lambert (eds), *Psychotherapy Relationships that Work,* Vol. 1: *Evidence-Based Therapist Contributions* (pp. 167–204). Oxford University Press.

Wampold, B.E. (2019). *The Basics of Psychotherapy: An Introduction to Theory and Practice* (2nd ed.). American Psychological Association.

Wampold, B.E. & Fluckiger, C. (2023). The alliance in mental health care: Conceptualization, evidence and clinical applications. *World Psychiatry, 22*(1), 25–41.

Wampold, B.E. & Imel, Z.E. (2015). *The Great Psychotherapy Debate: The Evidence for What Makes Psychotherapy Work* (2nd ed.). Routledge Taylor & Francis Group.

Wampold, B.E., Mondin, G.W., Moody, M., Stich, F., Benson, K., & Ahn, H. (1997). A meta-analysis of outcome studies comparing bona fide psychotherapies: Empirically, "All must have prizes." *Psychological Bulletin, 122*(3), 203–215.

Watson, J.C. (2007). Reassessing Rogers' necessary and sufficient conditions of change. *Psychotherapy, 44*(3), 268–273.

Zhang, A., Franklin, C., Currin-McCulloch, J., Park, S., & Kim, J. (2018). The effectiveness of strength-based, solution-focused brief therapy in medical settings: A systematic review and meta-analysis of randomized controlled trials. *Journal of Behavioral Medicine, 41*(2), 139–151.

3 The Influence of a Humanistic, Solution-Focused Approach on Healthcare Research

Laura R. Bowman

Background/Context

I am a researcher with a clinical background in occupational science and occupational therapy. In both cases, the term "occupation" refers to how people meaningfully and purposefully occupy (or spend, devote, engage in) their time. Specifically, I am a qualitative and clinically oriented researcher with a focus on transitions, lived experiences, and social engagement within a paediatric rehabilitation hospital. My area of focus is transitions throughout and out of paediatric care for children, youth, and their families. In my roles, I work with diverse groups of individuals (different age groups, sectors, roles, and agendas/goals). Through my work, I seek to understand how people experience and make meaning of the world in which they operate, what they are hoping to accomplish, and the different elements that impact their ability to achieve their goals.

With a practice so intimately tied to the human experience and how people choose/are able to engage in their own lives, I was naturally drawn to the solution-focused (SF) approach. The philosophies and skills shared through the SFHCC program provided tangible and accessible practices through which I could implement my client-centred, resiliency-focused explorations of the human experience (e.g., questions, language, outlooks). The approach and philosophy have helped me move through projects (both research and clinical) with an acknowledgement of the problems being faced (keeping one foot in acknowledgement) and move forward with what can make a difference (one foot in possibility). It has moved me towards what I think of as a solution-focused research process, which I will describe in this chapter.

Experiences During the Year-Long Program

I remain grateful for the opportunity to integrate my SF knowledge throughout the different areas of my career and life (e.g., in moderating meetings, in mentoring staff and students, in honing my focus on what is working in life, in parenting my own children). One of the greatest areas of change following my participation in the SFHCC program was my approach to the research process, including development, design, and implementation. With each passing lesson and session, I gained

DOI: 10.4324/9781003414490-4

new and deeper insights into the nuanced, complex, and yet extremely logical SF approach. As I began implementing the tools and principles in my own context, I was (and remain to this day) shocked at how much they support effective communication and movement towards logical and contextually relevant solutions. As I mentioned, I apply these principles throughout my many life roles, and will focus on the research process applications in this chapter.

The Difference My Participation in the SFHCC Program Has Made

As a researcher situated within a clinical context, I strive to support an ecologically and data-driven approach to care (such as the value-creating learning health systems approach outlined by Menear et al., 2019); which means, I use the multiple data available to inform how client care and services are offered. Such an approach allows me to be meaningfully integrated into a healthcare team, and to work with the service providers, administrators, clients, and inter-agency partners to consider and decide what information is needed to best understand and inform which services are available, when, how, and with which meaningful outcomes. So much information … and from so many sources! This, in part, means that my role includes creating space for the multiplicity of agendas, needs, ideas, and outcomes that our many contributors need from research and knowledge translation projects. It also allows me to guide our group towards realistic solutions – a perfect inroad for a solution-focused process.

A solution-focused approach to our research process also fits with my team's and organization's general strengths-based approach to care. This approach, however, tends to sit at odds with the primarily problem-focused world of academia and, as such, I was faced with an opportunity to consider how we might take a strengths-focused approach to exploring client, family, clinician, and systems-level experiences in paediatric transitions while also acknowledging (and working *with*) the problems, systemic barriers, and challenges. Most importantly, my SFHCC background helped me to consider how we could do all this and move towards meaningful and preferred futures for the multiple actors involved.

As I delved further into the SF literature, the alignment and potential of the SF approach with my own ideal research process became increasingly striking. Specifically, it allowed for the coexistence, and complementary consideration of, the strengths-focused approach that is prized by my teams and organization, inclusion of contextually relevant considerations that are needed from a critical perspective, and the harnessing of local expertise and "what is already working" that is needed from a healthcare and program adoption perspective. Harnessing the alignment between the types of exploratory and experientially based research that I oversee and the solution-focused ethos, it seemed as though integrating SF practices into our broader research process would be natural. Specifically, I facilitated the integration of solution-focused processes into three areas of my research practice: (1) team communication and idea generation; (2) research design and construction; and (3) data collection/generation.

Team Communication and Idea Generation

As is explored throughout this book's previous chapters, an SF approach can help build a team's collective momentum towards their goals. I think of this as an extended exercise in "contracting," given that it is the team's opportunity to get to know one another's perspectives on what needs to happen for our project to be successful, and collectively consider what will be different once we have the knowledge. Guided by this line of thinking, we gather perspectives, consider what we want to know, what we *already* know, and what we are *already managing* to do to address the problem. We work together to craft a question and/or goal that is achievable and will yield meaningful and contextually relevant results.

As the facilitator of these conversations, I work with our contributors to consider what will be most helpful from the research. I usually divide this process into two guiding areas of discussion that align with the general SF process, being a discussion of the possibility, and an acknowledgement of constraints. The discussion of possibility will include questions about what we do know and what we *want* to know. This may look like the following:

When the project is complete:

What will we know that we do not know now?
What will we have that we do not have now?
What do we imagine as a product/outcome?
What will we be doing differently?

Our diverse research contributors tend to offer information that is unique to their fields as well as complementary to reaching their shared research goals. In these discussions, I use variations of the miracle question, exception question, amplification, and indirect complimenting to help the team collaboratively explore the potential of our area of inquiry.

I then guide the discussion towards acknowledgement of the problems, barriers, and limitations that are *aligned with* (and not exclusive of) the above-mentioned goals and strengths. When setting research goals and developing protocols that meet the multiple agendas of clinicians, researchers, administrators, client/family representatives, community collaborators, and funders, the ability to hold space for problems is essential. The ability to acknowledge limitations or barriers while simultaneously working with the team to consider "what has worked" or reminding them that the target issues "are not problematic at 100% intensity for 100% of the time," allows us to collectively identify areas for potentially fruitful inquiry or intervention. This might include exception questions, scaling exercises, and considerations around the concept of "good enough" for the timeframe of the proposed research project.

As an example of how this might look, we recently started a research relationship with a large organization. We were hoping to build a partnership that would span multiple research initiatives over four years. We hosted an introductory meeting with the new group. Rather than start the meeting with our own objectives, we posed the following SF questions to get to know one another:

- With the combination of our teams' knowledge and person-power, what can we learn/achieve that we are not doing now?
- When we meet again in one year, what will be happening that will show us that our collaboration is "successful"?
- In five years, when the project is complete and was wildly successful, what will be different for you?

These are just some of the questions we used to explore the shared goals and set a shared agenda for upcoming research initiatives. With this information, we were able to build a collaborative research agenda based on a shared vision of a preferred future, rather than the outcomes of a single study. Feedback from the new organization was that they had never held a meeting like that before, and they felt that the depth of information shared through the introductory SF questions allowed us all to cut right to the synchronicities of our work so that we could move forward while holding and honouring one another's visions.

Research Design and Construction

Once the ideas have been generated (and "contracted," preferably using the SF approach to the research process), details on the design and construction of the project itself must be undertaken. I note here that, as with any of the information in this book, the SF approach is meant to amplify the research process. The information given here is by no means a crash-course in research design, coordination, or management.

When designing and constructing a research project or program of research, consideration of audience is important and must be undertaken upfront. Regardless of epistemological roots, voice and perspective always influence whose solutions are presented and how they are represented. That is to say even the most "positivist" of projects originates based on the political, social, or cultural interests of those funding and conducting the research, and is therefore not a neutral and unquestioned "truth." In an SF research process, it is helpful to make the contributing perspectives explicit for yourself, so that we can know how and to whom the research will have to be accountable. The figure below presents a few examples of the different levels at which perspectives are impacted via interest, funding, cultural interest, or political agendas. These audiences represent both the constraints of the types of questions that can be asked (i.e., do they align with the multiple audiences' agendas?) and *for whom* the results will need to be meaningful.

I note here that constraints are not a negative thing, and neither is the politics behind answering to the various, hierarchical research audiences. These are simply realities in which we have to work to move science, knowledge, and collective action forward. Making these things explicit for yourself and your team will allow you to work within the necessary constraints to make changes that *are* possible right now, and only focus on what *can* be addressed in the current opportunity. These types of power hierarchies are more often made explicit in critically leaning research, and they can be important and helpful to reflect upon for all studies. Transparency regarding the actors and beneficiaries of research is not meant as a criticism; it is meant to help research teams consider the needs, desires, and preferred future outcomes for the various audiences. To assist in this process, helpful questions might include:

Preferred Future	When our research is successful, what will be different? *For whom?*
Strengths Focus	What do we already know/do well? How have we managed to explore this or similar topics in the past? How have we moved forward, even a little bit?
Exception Focus	Despite the outlined problems and barriers, how have we managed to explore and grow towards similar goals in the past?
Lead with Constraints, Good Enough	Given our current grant period/goal, what would be good enough to learn/propose *for this project*?

I have found that in my SF research process, being able to question the research process itself has been particularly revealing. This has been especially relevant in research that proposes to be client-centred or client-partnered (e.g., research that involves power-sharing and balancing claims of client-centredness with funder needs and organizational direction). From an SF foundational perspective, we consider people to be innately whole and to hold the solutions to their problems within themselves. This becomes more nuanced when we consider broader cultural or systemic problems such as healthcare access and deep-seated stigma. When we make claims of conducting "client-centred" or "patient-centred" research in healthcare, people mean many different things. Exercises like the chart and questions in Figure 3.1 and the list above can help researchers to consider *whose* voices and experiences are being represented in the research and remove or reduce the implication that the answer lies in the client to solve the "client's" problems that are actually manifestations of broader societal issues. Again, this is to say that we can address client issues and use

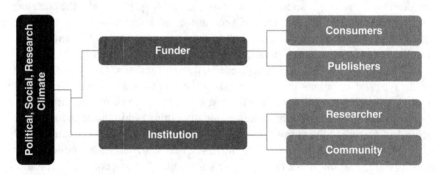

Figure 3.1 Research audiences

a client-informed approach; however, with an SF research process, we need deeper consideration of whose solutions they are and who must be involved in discovering and implementing them.

When constructing a research proposal and designing a research process, applying a SF research approach can also be helpful in identifying possible synergistic outcomes, and in determining what can reasonably be achieved with the given constraints for the multiple invested players. This clarity, when evaluated and considered regularly, has allowed me and my team to produce research proposals that are reasonable and harness the strengths of our team and our partners, while also considering the broader context in which the research will be conducted. These and other SF questions can be posed to/about research questions and methods (collection, analysis, dissemination) to help researchers consider whether they are on a fruitful path, and what might be different – and for whom – when the research is successful.

Data Collection/Generation

This is the area where researchers most commonly integrate SF approaches through SF language in interview questions (in qualitative research). While this is only one way in which to integrate the SF approach (of the many possibilities outlined above), it is a more common and powerful one. Indeed, SF communication can be helpful in the research process given that it:

- aligns with constructivist, interpretivist, and action-based research (if that is what you are using);
- allows for exploration of solutions and *what works* for research participants as they address problems; and
- facilitates a more shared power dynamic and an acknowledgement of different knowers (researcher, participant).

There are many benefits to using SF language for research interviews, and the process can open up meaningful and introspective dialogue – a win for experientially based research! We must, however, recall SF dialogue's therapeutic origins.

Using SF questions can lead to deep sharing on the part of research participants. Research interviews can be *therapeutic* for participants. A word of caution that researchers must be mindful that research questions are (usually) not intended to be *therapy*. Therapeutic interactions are outside of the scope of most research studies. It is important for researchers to know their own limits in any situation. This can be tricky, given that the intervention in solution focused coaching/brief therapy is the question, so how can we distinguish between a therapeutic question (intervention) and a research question (data-generation method)? Due to the nuanced nature of the SF coaching approach, it is difficult to give static examples of the differences between coaching and research questions. On the surface, the questions may look the same, but their function and intent may be different. It may be helpful to remember that when coaching, an SF practitioner will ask questions to delve deep, follow threads, and work towards personal solutions; when conducting research, an

SF practitioner will ask questions using SF language to promote deep thought on the research topic while the conversational flow follows a research interview guide (rather than the participant's own answers).

The Distinction between Coaching as a Therapeutic Experience, and SF Processes in Research

Interviewing is particularly important for the types of healthcare research that we conduct. When conducting research in the healthcare field, participants often discuss the most difficult areas of their lives, often caused by factors beyond their control. SF tools such as leading with constraints and using exception frames can help participants explore solutions while acknowledging personal, environmental, cultural, and systemic boundaries, but researchers must be careful not to promise outcomes or large-scale change when clients participate. There need to be firm expectations set on the limits of research outcomes/solutions.

The Difference an SF Approach Contributes to Healthcare in General

Beyond the outcomes of individual coaching sessions, an SF approach helps to facilitate collaboration towards solutions. By that I mean that – despite a historical problem-focus – teams of collaborators that include and value expertise from medical/health perspectives as much as lived experience of health or disability, program administration, funding and policy, and other relevant fields can work together on solutions that mutually consider one another's needs and agilely accommodate one another. This humanistic approach to a human-centred industry is both a nice and necessary way to operate that promotes collaboration and effective use of resources that are *already* available and working. I feel that this approach is refreshing for teams who are used to fighting their constraints rather than accepting and building creatively within them.

Favourite Tools and Principles

With so many great tools to work with, I find myself drawn to the principle that "the absence of something is not a goal." This resonates with me in a field where my currency is questions and goals (research), and an industry that is focused on reducing resources including time, personnel, and funding (healthcare). Remembering that the absence of something (resource, pain, bad experiences) is not a helpful goal to work toward, and allows me an in-road to start a SF process in developing a team's goal and amplifying our collective momentum.

Reference

Menear, M., Blanchette, M.A., Demers-Payette, O., & Roy, D. (2019). A framework for value-creating learning health systems. *Health Research Policy and Systems, 17*(1), 1–13.

4 How Solution-Focused Conversations Changed My Practice

A Reflection on the Synergy of Bioethics Consults and a Solution-Focused Approach

Dolly Menna-Dack

Sitting in my office across from a hard-working, dedicated healthcare provider during an ethics consult, I realized, a miracle happened. It did not happen overnight as the Miracle Question may have you believe; it was a slow build up, a layering of sorts. I was enrolled in the Solution-Focused Health Care Coaching program (SF-HCC) at Holland Bloorview Kids Rehabilitation Hospital and had been dutifully attending my classes for many weeks, trying out what I was learning, playing with the concepts, consciously re-framing my approach to lead from behind. And then one day I realized a miracle happened.

I have had a long and deep relationship with the health care system; I assume many of you have as well. You might be a healthcare provider, an administrator, a volunteer, a learner, a scientist, a client, or a family member. You may be many of those things, and you might even be none. Maybe you are connected to the healthcare system in way that I have not named; I would believe that because there are so many roles that support both the healthcare system and the delivery of each individual healthcare interaction. I notice that the further I get into my career, the more contemplative I become. Lately, I have struggled to answer the question: Is the business of a hospital to deliver healthcare to individual people, or is it to provide the structures that make the delivery of each and every single healthcare intervention possible? And because I continue to ponder this question, I can't help but perceive the vast importance of the many roles we all play in this system.

I became a bioethicist because I was and am still deeply interested in how children and families navigate healthcare decision-making. Yes, I work in paediatrics – I am interested in how adults using the health system make care decisions as well, and yet, the nuance of children, teens, and their loved ones really sparks my interest. You see there is something a bit different about children and teens – they live in the realm of learning, of feedback, mistakes, self-discovery, and solution-finding. These things are ever-present in their lives. Children and youth are paying attention, they are working from a place of values they have learned from close relationships and influences, and they test and try out what they have learned, they develop their own values, and they keep what they like and discard what doesn't work for them.

DOI: 10.4324/9781003414490-5

We, as a society, acknowledge this process as "growing up"; we make choices, experience joys and disappointments, and we learn. We learn what works for us and we try to do more of what works, especially if it leads to an outcome we want.

You may remember a time in your youth where you desired something enough that you eventually found a solution to get what you wanted. Perhaps you wanted a later bedtime, so you showed your family you could wake up independently and not be cranky and overtired; maybe you wanted to buy something, so you did chores for an allowance, got a paper route, or babysat the neighbours' kids. As children and teens, we are constantly finding out what works and using what we learn in other, similar situations.

Because children and teens are constantly going through this process, parents and caregivers go through it as well. Adults learn what works for their own kids, they become deeply proficient at reading a glance, sigh, or wail from their child, and they try options to see what answers, comforts, or activities soothe them. Ever seen an adult with a fussing baby? The adult is focused on trying to invent a way to settle that baby and the moment they find that the baby is even just a little bit more settled – they do more of it! And, in my own experience, parents are ready to share with all would-be baby-holders just what to do to keep their baby happy and settled. They don't waste time filling you in on what not to do. It's like a football play and they are the quarterback with the clock still running: Blue blanket! Small bottle! Squeeze her tight! You've got precious seconds and none to waste on things that don't work.

So why does the dynamic of paediatric healthcare decision-making interest me so much? Well, for some children, they will continue to need support to make their healthcare decisions for their whole life, even as adults, while some children can and want to participate in healthcare decision-making to the fullest extent that they are able to from the moment they become clients of the healthcare system. I like the range that exists in paediatrics, and I acknowledge that childhood disability, neurodiversity, personal experience, and family context (among others) will all impact the emerging autonomy of children and teens. I won't lie, I also really enjoy teens with "typical teen attitudes," the ones who some may not bother trying to engage, the ones who look like they'd rather be anywhere else in the world at that moment. But I get that, who wouldn't want to be somewhere else rather than receiving healthcare?

Have you met a bioethicist before? Are you a bioethicist? More often than not, I find myself answering "What is bioethics?" and "So, what do you do as a bioethicist?" I like the Joint Center for Bioethics at the University of Toronto's answer to this question:

> … bioethics is about the values each of us bring – as a patient, family member, clinician, administrator, scientist, policymaker, or citizen – to our experience of health and the health system. It is also about what to do when our values conflict, whose values matter in a decision, or how to make a decision if there is uncertainty or more than one possible "right answer."
>
> (JCB, 2022)

This answer sums it up; in a health system where science and technology continue to advance, our own personal values and, in some cases, the values of our community and society, bioethics indeed plays a role in helping us to decide what is best given the possible options. Bioethicists seek to support those making healthcare decisions, those offering healthcare choices, and those working, volunteering, and learning in the structures and systems related to healthcare.

As a paediatric bioethicist, I am involved in many discussions about "best interests" and what is in the best interest of the child. Who is the one deciding? Is the child able to make this decision; is the child able to make smaller decisions that are related to this big decision? How do we explain the decision in a way the family, let alone the child, will understand? Another line of discussion that fits like an old glove is about children's rights to privacy and their desire to have some of it! Imagine a gaggle of health professionals communicating with you, making notes, and sharing it all with your family; it doesn't feel like there is much opportunity for choice, for control, or for decision-making, does it? And so, we engage in conversations about children's rights; their rights to choose, their rights to privacy, and the importance of respecting them both as a member of a family and as a unique individual who is in the process of growing up.

Since my work is largely based in conversation, I surmised the way to become an even better bioethicist was to hone my conversation skills. I have sought out courses that focus on specific skills. For example, conflict management was fun, although for one of my class assignments, a group project, my professor told me that I had not followed the directions for assignment. My role in the group was to role play the mediator. I was tasked with getting my classmates to come to a compromise on the height of a backyard fence and a construction timeline. My assignment was to mediate until 50% of the overall outcome was agreed on and then stop the proceedings. Using the newly taught techniques, I quickly engaged the two "neighbours" in an exercise to discuss what could be done. I stated something has to be done, so let's figure it out. At the end of our allotted time, my "neighbours" were shaking hands; they had agreed on the height of the fence and the construction timeline, and I truly believe that if they had really been neighbours, they would have made plans for a backyard BBQ once the work was completed. However, my professor was not impressed. "You missed the point of the assignment," he told me. "You were supposed to get them to compromise, not agree." All these years later, I still do not understand why my result wasn't A+ work; my groupmates had agreed – even if I missed the point of the assignment. I had facilitated a conversation where they were able to find solutions that worked for both of them. In the end, I wasn't dissuaded; I still wanted to enhance my conversation skills.

In mid-2020 at the height of the COVID-19 pandemic, I received an email request from Dr Elaine Cook, worded so: "The Solution-Focused Health Care Coach program has been approved for national accreditation, which is super exciting" (E. Cook, personal communication, May 5, 2020). Elaine went on to explain her request, that the program would need a Code of Ethics, one that would acknowledge the uniqueness of the dualities and responsibilities that the healthcare providers who would become graduates of the new program would need to recognize, to respect, and to deftly navigate. I was intrigued and excited to bring the ethics lens to the newly accredited program. The development of the code of ethics took me on a journey that included an environmental scan, reviewing literature, and conversations with Elaine and her initial cohort of participants. I am proud to say that the Solution Focused Health Care Coaching Code of Ethics is a part of the manual and is governing document for the program offered at Holland Bloorview Kids Rehabilitation Hospital. The code is clear, it is simple, and it creates a space that acknowledges the potential duality of the role of the coach while honouring a solution-focused stance. The guiding principles are Quality, Safety, Humility, Autonomy, and Respect (Holland Bloorview Kids Rehabilitation Hospital, n.d.).

Almost two years later, I was a graduate of the Solution-Focused Health Care Coach program and by that time the miracle had happened. Like a good student, I had been trying out what I was learning, in my private life, not my professional life (at first). In fact, my peer coach (a dear friend and colleague of mine) and I convinced my mother to let us practise on her. We co-coached, in the beginning stopping and starting, trying to pick up the thread of the conversation, sometimes breaking out into peels of laughter when one of us "opened the wrong door." Afterwards, we quizzed my mother about what worked and then we sat and reflected about our next steps. Over time, things got a little smoother, and our approaches started to shift. I moved on to coaching my younger brother once a week while I was in the program. He's a good guy my little brother, you might be able to tell that we are a family that is supportive of one another's quest for new knowledge, we are partial to coaching, and we believe that goals can be set and achieved. Basically, I could not have asked for a better test environment for practising my new skills and no other environment would have so clearly forced me to come up against my own habits: like my deep love of the role of older sister who is ready to give advice, and "suggest" exactly *how* it should be accomplished and *when* it should be accomplished! My time in the course was fun and as my comfort level grew and my conversation skills enhanced, I soon started to use a solution-focused approach at work.

There are multiple tenets of the solution-focused approach that map readily onto bioethics practice. For example, the idea of contracting with a client and leading with constraints is an important element of informed consent. Be clear – tell the client what they can expect, ask what they want, get consent to start. Respecting the autonomy of the client, recognizing that they are experts in their own lives, and believing that they can find their own solutions aligns the fundamental concepts of patient- and family-centred care. The Institute of Patient and Family Centered Care (IPFCC) highlights that "a key goal is to promote the health and well-being of individuals and families and to maintain their control" (IPFCC, n.d.).

Clarity, agreement, check-ins, these solution-focused coaching tools are all consistent with the guiding principles of Respect and Autonomy found in the program's code of ethics. "Good enough" is basically the day-to-day work of a bioethicist. If you remember, the Joint Centre for Bioethics points out that bioethics is concerned with "how to make a decision if there is uncertainty or more than one possible 'right answer'" exists and let me tell you, sometimes the option or choice that is "good enough" is the best possible option in a given situation.

The Institute for Patient and Family Centered Care states that "patient- and family-centered care is working 'with' patients and families, rather than just doing 'to' or 'for' them" (IPFCC, n.d.) and then goes on to say, "a key goal is to promote the health and well-being of individuals and families and to maintain their control." To me, this description begs the question: How can you possibly be providing patient- and family-centred care if you are not using a solution-focused approach?

The view is better when you lead from behind. When you lead from the front, you don't actually know if the other person is following, they could have gotten lost, saw something they found to be more important, or started on a new path, and you wouldn't even know. When you lead from behind, you can confirm that you are going in the direction that the consultee wants to go. When you lead from behind, instead of pulling someone along a path that you are actively choosing, you instead "embrace the role of the coach and allow the client's voice, wisdom, and choice to be central" (SFHCC Code of Ethics, 2020) and, if you do, you might just realize when a miracle happens.

Take a breath, get comfortable, and imagine me sitting in my office across from a hard-working, dedicated healthcare provider during an ethics consult.

I have invited this healthcare provider in and closed the door so that we can have a private conversation. I have asked if this time still works for them. "Yes," they reply. "Have you had a busy day today?" I ask. "Yes," they reply. "Would you like to talk about the situation?" "Yes," they reply. The "Yes Set" is another solution-focused tool that I have found to be effective in quickly building rapport, signalling that the ethics consult is about to start and demonstrating that the consultee is in control: they are the ones choosing to have the ethics consult and deciding if we can go ahead.

"Ok," I say. I give the limits of confidentiality, and slip easily into asking how, in the next 30 minutes, I can be most helpful to them. Our conversation proceeds, I offer acknowledgements and compliments because they are easy to spot, and this provider's dedication and moral distress are equally easy to identify. And then we get to the heart of the issue.

I asked my colleague to imagine, to imagine they went home and there was no traffic, dinner was cooked and waiting for them, and, if you can believe it, the house was also tidy. I asked them to imagine that they went to bed and slept through the night, having a restful sleep, and that this issue they came to see me about did not keep them up or wake them up. I told them that while they were sleeping, a miracle happened. Then, I asked them to tell me what they might notice, when they awoke in the morning, that would tell them this miracle had happened. What would be different for them? And that's when I realized a miracle really did happen.

I set out to become an even better bioethicist, to hone my conversation skills. And in this moment, I realized that the integration of solution-focused tools in my practice had made me an even better bioethicist and the skill that I had honed was my ability to listen and ask good questions that help individuals find their own meaningful solutions.

References

Holland Bloorview Kids Rehabilitation Hospital. (n.d.). Solution Focused Health Care. Coaching Code of Ethics. Available at: https://s3.amazonaws.com/kajabi-storefronts-production/sites/163318/themes/2151380827/downloads/7gVB6ovWTcGLVbxAGYLQ_HCSFC_Code_of_Ethics_09-2020.pdf

Institute for Patient- and Family-Centered Care. (n.d.). Patient- and family-centred care. Available at: https://www.ipfcc.org/about/pfcc.html

Joint Center for Bioethics. (2022). What is bioethics? Available at: https://jcb.utoronto.ca/bioethics-in-action/what-is-bioethics/

Section Two

Clinical Applications

5   A Solution-Focused Approach for Healthcare Providers Supporting Autistic Children and Youth

Moira Peña

"We don't look at a calla lily, and say it has a 'petal deficit disorder,' we appreciate its beautiful shape."

Dr Thomas Armstrong, Executive Director of
the American Institute for Learning

"Becoming a solution focused clinician can be learned, much as a new language is acquired."

Anne Bodmer Lutz, MD

As a paediatric occupational therapist, I work with autistic children to support the various "occupations" or daily tasks of childhood, including those that they may want or need to do at school. In order to assess handwriting skills, for example, I may ask children to colour in a picture and, while they are engaging in that task, I observe and collect information to then hypothesize as to what may be getting in the way of their success. As a healthcare professional working within the medical system, I've been trained to be particularly adept at identifying differences that situate the child outside of what is considered to be typical development – that is, I immediately notice and assess deficits of what the child "can't do."

I started colouring a picture of an elephant in grey and gave Johnny*, a 7-year-old autistic child, his own copy of the drawing. I then pointed to a colouring set he could use. He started the task and I proceeded to use my well-honed deficit lens to immediately notice every single thing that Johnny did "wrong" – the unconventional way in which he held his pencil, the uncommon hard pressure he placed on it, the atypical intonation he used when he spoke, the times he coloured outside the lines, the difficulties he had with looking at me or "maintaining eye contact" while interacting with me. I even remember thinking to myself that his visual skills might have been affected as I noticed that he was colouring his elephant in *pink*. I added this observation to my already long list of "deficits" and decided to delve further. "Johnny," I asked him, "what is the colour of elephants?" "Grey," he clearly said without looking up from his paper. I then asked: "Johnny, what colour is your elephant?" "Pink," he responded. I looked at him in confusion and proceeded to slow down my rate of speech and enunciate clearly (common therapist behaviour

DOI: 10.4324/9781003414490-7

when we don't get immediate compliance to our requests and therefore we begin to make assumptions about the person's capacity for understanding) and then asked: "So Johnny, why is your elephant pink?" Without missing a beat, he responded, "because this elephant is sunburnt."

I was rendered momentarily speechless, laughed for a few seconds and then proceeded to *really* look at him. And in that moment, I saw it *all* – his humour, his delightful curious nature, his creativity, his resourcefulness, the way in which his manner of speaking punctuated certain sounds which served for me to pay full attention to his communication – in other words, I saw and *appreciated* his differences, realized that these could be reframed as personal strengths, and became keenly aware that the person who needed changing was (dare I say it!) *me.*

This was the beginning of my (ongoing!) journey towards shifting my practice (and that of other therapists learning from me), from one that focuses solely on pathology and remediation to one in which steps are explicitly taken towards adopting solution-focused and strengths-based approaches instead. Work long enough in the system and one slowly but surely begins to realize that the value of our therapeutic interventions (and of ourselves as therapists!) is tied to how close our therapy outcomes are to matching the autistic child's skills to those of neurotypical children. In other words, how effective are we as therapists in changing this child to make them indistinguishable from their neurotypical peers? This recognition prompted some soul searching as I reflected on a key solution-focused question we often ask in our sessions with our clients and families: W*hat is it that I wanted instead?* And the answer became impossible to continue to ignore: I wanted a practice that was centred on validating and amplifying capabilities and strengths that were already there and that honoured a person's full humanity irrespective of the body (and mind!) that was apparent.

The question becomes, how do we begin to make this shift in a world that prefers non-disabled ways of being? We begin by recognizing that our healthcare role involves not only noticing and addressing challenges that come with a diagnosis, but also holds identifying and leveraging strengths – within our clients, within their families or key people supporting them, and within ourselves – *in equal value.* Being intentional about using a solution-focused and strengths-based lens is hard work as it calls for healthcare professionals to come face to face with personal and professional biases, question deeply ingrained beliefs around disability, and engage in a process of (mostly) unlearning. Adopting this lens can also be incredibly rewarding, however, as it honours a paradigm shift that is already taking place in autism care and empowers occupational therapists (and other healthcare professionals) to confidently practise in a way that truly aligns with our humanistic and client-centred values.

Here are three steps, with accompanying key solution-focused questions, that healthcare providers can use to begin that journey:

1 **Take time to reflect on and identify professional and personal biases:** We all have implicit biases, feelings, and attitudes that we may not be fully aware of and it is important to explore these as they can negatively affect the ways

in which we conduct assessments, develop care plans, and even interact with our clients. The medical field has a long history of viewing disabled people as "abnormal," of associating differences with weaknesses, and of making negative assumptions about disability in general. If we are only deficit-focused in our approach, however, we can have some unintended harmful consequences for people whose developmental and physical trajectories differ from the norm. For example, we may make negative assumptions around a person's cognitive capacity based on their degree of observable motor involvement. An autistic person who is constantly in rocking motion is often assumed to be someone with diminished cognitive capacity when, in fact, research has uncovered that motor movement may be outside of an autistic person's willful control and may therefore be unrelated to the person's cognitive abilities. By *making positive assumptions and presuming competence instead*, we are then able to consider that the autistic person may not be able to use spoken language as a form of communication (a task that requires a high degree of motor involvement), but may be able to communicate using an augmentative and alternative communication (AAC) device. Once we identify and address our biases and begin to view different forms of communication as equally valuable, we are then more able to explore possibilities and collaborate with other service providers, the client, and the family to explore all available forms of communication.

Key solution-focused questions we can reflect on to begin to address personal and professional biases are:

- Is this (assessment, intervention, report) strengths-based, meaningful, and of value to the client and/or family I am collaborating with?
- Suppose that what I am doing is meaningful and valuable to the client and/or their family, what difference might that make to the client, their family, and to myself as a clinician?
- What will I be doing differently that will show my clients and/or their families that I am becoming aware of my biases and taking steps to address them?
- How will I notice that I am progressing in taking these steps? What will others notice?

2 **Practise being curious and remain open to learning from your clients' (and their families') lived experience:** Adopting a solution-focused and strengths-based lens means moving away from our long-held "expert" stance where we as healthcare providers have all the answers. Instead, we recognize that our clients and their families are the experts of their own lives and we become collaborative partners in their healthcare journeys. This means that we learn from the community we are serving, which, in my world, means learning from autistic people. Autistic adults are asking healthcare professionals to see beyond pathology and recognize that differences or variations in neurological development and functioning across human beings can be viewed as natural and even valuable aspects of the human condition. Each person's autism then informs their unique autistic identity and, as such, we as healthcare providers are being called upon to embrace and promote the acceptance of autistic and authentic ways of

being. We begin by maintaining a stance of curiosity with our clients and their families, asking questions and staying present while listening to their unique stories, and relating to them as equals. In this way, we work alongside the client and their family to ensure that therapy prioritizes achieving what they want their preferred future to be.

Solution-focused questions we can begin to include in our conversations to adopt a stance of curiosity while remaining open to learning from our clients and their families are:

- What will my clients and their families notice that will show them that I am present in our conversation and listening to their unique narratives?
- What will others notice in my reports that will show them that I am valuing my clients' lived experiences and the voices of the autistic community?
- What will my clients and families notice that I am doing differently as I begin to take this step towards adopting solution-focused and strengths-based approaches in my practice?

3 **Use language that inspires a future focus and a sense of agency in your clients and their families:** It is important to notice the language we use when interacting with clients and their families because our words inform and shape our perceptions. "Words generate our worlds," says Joshua Heschel, and, as such, adopting solution-focused and strengths-based approaches in our practices means that we carefully choose and make explicit use of language that inspires hope and a sense of agency in our clients and/or their families. In this way, our healthcare conversations become therapeutic tools in and of themselves that enable us to shift our focus from a conversation solely discussing problems (what we don't want) to one that moves towards identifying and amplifying solutions (what we want). This process includes noticing and amplifying what our clients and families are already doing well, using respectful and identity-affirming language, while also supporting them in identifying what steps (however small) they can take towards their preferred future. In this way, our clients and their families become active participants in the therapy process as they are the ones who determine how they will move forward towards their preferred futures with our support.

Solution-focused questions we can begin to include in our conversations to inspire hope and a sense of agency are:

- What are your best hopes for our time together? How will you know that this session would have been helpful?
- What does your child enjoy? What about them do you enjoy?
- What does it look like when your child is happy, relaxed, and engaged?
- Can you describe or tell me about moments when you've noticed that your child was already happy, relaxed, and engaged?
- What has worked for you in the past to help your child remain in a happy, relaxed, and engaged state?
- As difficult as it is, what are you noticing about yourself that tells you that you are already managing?

Adopting a solution-focused and strengths-based approach has enabled me to move from a narrative of "fixing and curing" to one that holds a more balanced and holistic view of a person, one that compels me to explicitly identify strengths, and not just those that reside within my clients, but also those that are present within their families and within ourselves as therapists. Engaging in solution-focused conversations has also provided me with a new worldview – one in which people's strengths and resources are amplified and their full human complexity is appreciated irrespective of the challenge (however significant!) they present with. A worldview that accepts and values differences and enables me to confidently practise in a manner that upholds what truly matters to my clients and their families.

References

Dallman, A.R., Williams, K.L., & Villa, L. (2022). Neurodiversity – affirming practices are a moral imperative for occupational therapy. *Open Journal of Occupational Therapy, 10*(2), 1–9.

Higashida, N. (2013). *The Reason I Jump: One Boy's Voice from the Silence of Autism.* Hachette.

Lutz, A.B. (2013). *Learning Solution-Focused Therapy: An Illustrated Guide.* American Psychiatric Publishing.

Sterman, J., Gustafson, E., Eisenmenger, L., Hamm, L., & Edwards, J. (2023). Autistic adult perspectives on occupational therapy for autistic children and youth. *Occupational Therapy Journal of Research, 43*(2), 237–244.

6 Dealing with Behaviour

Collaborative Behaviour Support

Heidi Schwellnus and Brian Freel

Holland Bloorview Kids Rehabilitation Hospital has had a solution-focused (SF) approach to healthcare for over ten years. This approach fits well with our Client and Family integrated approach to care (Law et al., 2003) because it encourages the clinical care team to focus on the strengths and resources of the client and family instead of the predominant problem-focused approach common in medicine (Baldwin et al., 2013). A second tenet of the SF approach that also fits well with client- and family-centred care is the recognition that the individual is the expert in their own lived experience and has the inherent ability to harness their strengths and resources to create their preferred outcome.

The hospital has a focus on physical habilitation and rehabilitation of children with congenital and acquired disabilities. In the pursuit of the client's and family's desired outcomes, there can be challenges in achieving full participation on behalf of the paediatric clients. This can take the form of challenging or interfering behaviours that can impact the achievement of the goals or the delay of that achievement, which results in longer stays, an outcome that is often not helpful for the family and can result in more expense to the hospital.

To manage these situations, the hospital had an established behaviour training system in place to support staff; however, the training tended to focus on significantly escalated situations. A working group promoted a framework that involved a three-step approach to managing behaviour (see Figure 6.1), with the existing training focused on the most escalated situations, or step 3. However, there was a belief among some leaders that a focus on prevention of escalations might enable staff to influence the outcome of the situation better and more positively. To assist with this, the hospital augmented the escalation training with behaviour guidance principles training. Staff learned to provide choices to clients, using a first this, then that approach. This basic training is now embedded into staff orientation. For step 2, leadership reviewed existing approaches to behaviour training, including the collaborative behaviour support (CBS) coaching model created by Elaine Cook, one of the editors of this book. The CBS model was selected from a range of training options because the principles and skills of the model are humanistic and solution-focused, which amplifies the SF work already being done within the organization, as well as provides a consistency of training many staff had already received. The CBS model was also the most flexible regarding training approach and adaptability

DOI: 10.4324/9781003414490-8

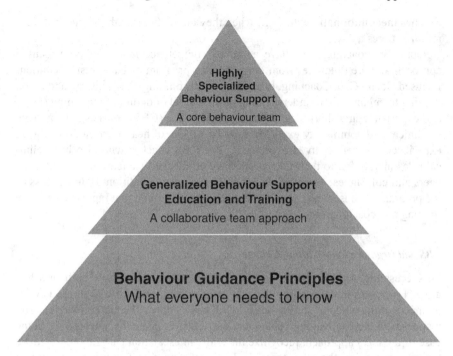

Figure 6.1 Behaviour Guidance Framework

and it built on existing staff expertise in solution-focused coaching. As a result, the training required for facilitators was minimal.

In this chapter, we will describe the CBS program. Heidi Schwellnus will provide details about the context and process of implementing the CBS program at Holland Bloorview Kids Rehabilitation Hospital, while Brian Freel will provide some experiential context as a CBS coach.

The Context and Implementation of the CBS Program

One of the key components of the CBS training model is the addition of one-on-one and group coaching for staff to support their implementation of the tools learned. The CBS facilitators are called CBS coaches and they round on the inpatient units to support staff in addressing the challenging behaviours of clients, meet with staff to find solutions when challenging situations occur, and assist in integrating the learnings into common everyday practice. This post-workshop coaching support has been supported in the literature to encourage more implementation of information from workshops after the fact (own peer coaching review). The coaches support the inpatient units 5 days per week, are part of behaviour "rounds" meetings where the team of nursing staff and others gather to discuss current challenging situations, and meet with staff formally during the education-focused workshops, which vary in length to suit the staff structure on each unit. In addition, the CBS coaches meet informally with staff, when they circulate through the medical units multiple times a day.

Our CBS coaching staff have achieved competence in the solution-focused approach and are graduates from our year-long program of Humanistic Solution-Focused Health Care Coaching. In addition to this training, they undergo additional training to enhance their understanding of the funnel of optimal functioning (FOF) and experience in a short-term coaching setting. The (CBS) coaches have a range of clinical and community experience, and a variety of health and non-healthcare experience, as well as lived experience. The CBS coaches who also have clinical roles in addition to their CBS work have established valued rapport with their peers and colleagues; however, this is not a necessary condition to the success of the program as those who are new to the organization build that rapport during the training and coaching sessions.

CBS and Organizational Culture Change

To successfully embed this model into practice requires a culture shift in a few areas. First is an understanding that the environment, and those in it, are key influencers of the outcome during behavioural interactions. The staff's reactions and responses to the challenging behaviours can either escalate the situation or, in the case of the CBS approach, recognize the shifts in escalation early and de-escalate the situation using the CBS tools, including the funnel of optimal functioning, which helps them to gauge where the client is regarding the escalation and select appropriate tools. A second culture shift is the notion or understanding that behaviour is a normal part of interactions with children and youth. Behaviour is a form of communication of wants and needs and must be acknowledged as communication. One of the key ingredients of this approach is a tool or framework that incorporates the FOF (Cook, 2022). Awareness of this tool is key regarding both the child/family and staff. The FOF amplifies observation and reflection skills, slowing down the default escalation response that is common in situations where staff feel uncertain or unsafe, or less competent that they might otherwise.

CBS Training

The training involves 4–6 hours of workshop attendance for staff, which is a sizeable time commitment to undertake. The initial design was arranged to suit nursing shift work and support the replacement staff to cover two nurses participating in the workshop over a one-day period. This approach has had a positive success rate in the past for education within the hospital. However, currently, with staffing challenges as well as many other pressing education items to be considered, the workshops have been adapted to 1 hour in length with four to six sessions in total. Breaking the training down into more manageable chunks has allowed for more flexible time management since backfill is no longer required and the information is shared with staff within their own units in a more informal setting. We currently offer a mix of these two approaches to our inpatient staff, as well as the potential for two or three 2-hour workshops to maximize the staff's ability to attend the sessions in challenging times.

As mentioned previously, one of the key additions to this education and training is the on-site CBS coaches who lead/facilitate the training sessions and provide in-the-moment coaching feedback to staff regarding interactions with clients and families. Coaching has been supported as a successful method to embed workshop learning into practice (Schwellnus & Carnahan, 2014). The CBS process is described later in this chapter.

Beyond the FOF as a key tool, the other significant and pivotal understanding that makes this approach so useful and effective is the understanding on the staff's part that their responses to a client's behaviour greatly impact the situation and outcomes associated with the situation, and they can influence those situations and outcomes with the principles and skills learned during the program. As a training aid, two simulation videos were created and are embedded into the training. In both videos, actors played the client/family who was escalating. For both actors, during the creation of the video, they were instructed to just respond as they felt appropriate to the responses from the staff in the situation; no knowledge of the techniques was shared. Two versions were recorded. The first version depicted the typical response of a staff member to a client/parent escalation. The staff members became escalated, were defensive and frustrated. The second version involved the CBS-trained staff responding to the client/parent escalation. Despite significant effort, neither the client nor the parent managed to escalate the trained staff; in fact, a level of engagement and rapport was built that enabled a transformative experience. These videos are fundamental components of the learning and demonstrate the impact of using the strategies in common situations. They are analyzed in ways that highlight the differences in response in both versions. This analysis is empowering for staff because it demonstrates how small dialogic and humanistic skills have a significant impact on the outcome of a situation.

The CBS Program Applied

While Heidi provided the context, rationale, and details of how Holland Bloorview came to invest in and adopt the CBS program, I (Brian) provide the experiential perspective, as one of the CBS coaches with three decades of community and private practice experience. Prior to becoming a graduate of the SFHCC program at Holland Bloorview, I worked in a variety of environments where individuals, in the care of professionals, were habitually exhibiting behaviours that were both disruptive and challenging, including: residential settings, formal educational settings, intense behaviour modification programs, lockdown facilities, and hospital psychiatric wards. In addition to these environments, I have worked with individuals with a host of behavioural and mental health challenges, including but not limited to, acquired brain injuries, autism spectrum disorder, oppositional defiant disorder, conduct disorder, alcoholism, drug addiction, suicidal behaviour, antisocial personality disorder, and psychopathic personality disorder. Initially, I was fortunate enough to simply observe other professionals as they interacted with many of these individuals – and their behaviours. Much of what I witnessed in my early days in this field resembled trial and error and patchwork. There were some boundaries and consistency, although I noticed there was little or no collaboration between staff and clients, and there was more of an us *against* them atmosphere. I remember thinking, it wasn't surprising that individuals don't work in this field very long or start showing signs of burnout quicker than most.

Something that intrigued me then, and still does today, is how each staff member interacted with and supported their clients. I found myself noticing subtle differences in these interactions with their clients and took note of the differing results these varying interactions and supports would yield. I quickly realized rapport and relationship-building were the most important factors that contributed to harmonious interactions. I was always looking at what contributed to rapport and relationship-building as well as how I/we could do this better, or differently. There wasn't much emphasis on rapport and relationship-building back then, so, of course, there were no instructions or training to help us achieve this with our clients. While keeping the importance of rapport and relationship-building in mind, I was still keenly interested in strategies that were effective regardless of who was implementing them or the relationship(s) that were established between staff and clients. Upon reflection, I realize I was looking for a universal method that focused more on interventions, where positive outcomes were a result of collaboration, as opposed to compliance.

The Collaborative Behaviour Support (CBS) Process

I currently work as a CBS coach and facilitator at Holland Bloorview Kids Rehabilitation Hospital. Heidi explained earlier in the chapter that this work involves supporting staff who are experiencing challenging behaviours with clients and family members. I am one of four CBS coaches who cover the hospital's three in-patient units. As CBS coaches, we provide an array of support services: one-on-one and group/team coaching sessions, observing staff members while they engage in procedures with clients who are identified as challenging because of their behaviours, real-time debriefs, and education and training.

CBS is a collaborative systems approach that creates positive care environments where care providers and clinicians have the knowledge, understanding, skills, and support to engage with clients in ways that *elicit, amplify, and reinforce strengths and resources* of the care provider and clinicians – as well as the client. CBS provides a number of tools/interventions that allow care providers to be curious while being supportive and helping them to move up the Funnel of Optimal Functioning (FOF). The CBS model is grounded in a solid understanding of the FOF. When clinicians and care providers learn to use the FOF to assess their client's functioning, the most appropriate response given the client's position is apparent. Clinicians become more successful engaging with clients and families, behaviour becomes less of a stress point, and, as a result, clinicians feel more competent and confident themselves.

As a result of our team's successes, it soon became clear that the work the CBS coaches were doing supported the work of our hospital's small behaviour support team. Our behaviour support process now begins with our Intake Team and in addition to our CBS coaches this team includes Youth Facilitators (intake screeners), Child Life Specialists/Child Youth Workers, and Board-Certified Behaviour Analysts (BCBAs). We refer to this as our Inpatient Behaviour Team (IBT).

This process starts with a brief Client Screening Questionnaire that provides the parents with an opportunity to share information about their child regarding such issues as important relationships, strengths, things their child enjoys doing, what helps them adapt to new environments, how they best express themselves, how they communicate pain or discomfort, what they don't like or what upsets them, how they may communicate that they are feeling anxious or upset, as well as what we can do to help them feel better when they are feeling anxious or upset. In addition, the parents are asked to share any other information that may help us to engage with and support their child. This usually takes about 10 minutes and provides us with valuable information that will assist us as we strive to build rapport and supportive relationships, which will enhance our ability to make the child's transition and stay at our facility as positive and productive as possible.

In the event that a potential challenging behaviour is identified, because of this Intake Questionnaire, the IBT is notified and discusses strategies as well as when the CBS coaches will contact and support staff. The CBS coaches will often make contact with the unit manager and frontline support staff, namely, nurses, therapists, etc., and inform them that they will be checking in periodically to offer ongoing support. At other times, staff or unit managers will reach out to the CBS coaches and request their support. This support is strengths-based and strategic in relation to eliciting staff's strengths, resources, what they are already doing well, and how they can do more of what is working, as well as what they would like to do differently in the future to enhance their working relationship(s) with their clients. A couple of examples of the impact our CBS coaches have had are described below.

Example 1

Something we do as CBS coaches to support staff who are finding a specific client exceptionally challenging is Observations & Debriefs. The staff will invite a CBS coach to observe them working with this challenging client. The coach will take notes related to what they see the staff doing as they work with the client. This provides the coach with some framework regarding the procedures the staff employs during their interactions with the client so the coach can ask specific questions related to what the staff member did well. For example, say the staff member is a physiotherapist and during the physiotherapy session the client struggles or refuses to do certain elements of the range of motion portion of the session. The coach can ask the staff what they believe they did well during that part of the physio session. The therapist will usually identify the part of the range of motion portion when the client was not struggling or refusing. This helps bring the therapist up the FOF and creates an opportunity for the coach to ask some probing and more challenging questions regarding what the therapist may do differently next time when they are working with this client to reduce the likelihood of the client struggling or refusing to do just a little more. The CBS coaches are equipped with several strategies to elicit positive responses and strengths from the therapists, and other staff, and will support the staff as they discuss ways to improve future interactions with their clients.

This is just a small example, although the staff we supported through this process are often surprised to be able to articulate several positive things they did well, especially when their typical assessment of the overall session may not have been positive. We often ask the staff to rate our Debriefs on a scale of 10–0, with 10 being very positive. They often share with the coaches that the experience was much more positive than they originally thought it would be and give a high rating number, usually 8 or 9 and sometimes a 10. This usually has the staff members asking the CBS coaches to attend more of their future sessions or interactions with clients.

Example 2

A team of staff members had a young male client who was growing increasingly challenging regarding his behaviour outbursts and had a recent incident where the client's behaviour turned physical, and a few staff members were injured. The unit manager invited the CBS coaches to attend a team meeting with the staff who were involved in the incident as well as other staff who were stressing over the potential of similar incidences occurring in the future. The meeting started with the staff who were present during the incident, explaining what happened and what they did that didn't work. The CBS coaches took a stance of curiosity and asked them to share just a few of the client's strengths and what the client enjoys doing.

The conversation quickly changed from the client's challenges and the problem(s) and the staff's concerns about working with this client in the future to a number of positive qualities the client already possessed. One staff member who was involved in the incident said, "He is actually quite a cute little guy." Other staff joined in and shared some admirable qualities this client possesses, as well as some positive interactions they'd recently had with this client. As the conversation progressed, the CBS coach asked about other experiences with this client that yielded positive outcomes. At this point, most, if not all, of the staff were sharing positive stories and strategies that had worked in the past. The two CBS coaches who attended this meeting were vigorously taking notes as the staff shared their stories and strategies that other staff members in the room had not considered that yielded positive outcomes for both the staff and the client.

The two coaches shared their notes with the unit manager the next day, who then shared the notes with their team to initiate some positive, impactful changes to support this client. The manager quickly replied to the coaches stating that changes were already happening and that they were amazed at the differences that were already noticeable in their staff, with just one small intervention. Over the next few days and weeks, the unit manager said they had fewer and fewer staff expressing to them their reluctance to work with this client.

A short time later, the unit manager nominated the entire behaviour support team for a Spotlight Recognition Award, which was granted to the team in recognition of compassion and excellence and for enhancing nursing care to this client with some challenging behaviours, and for helping the staff generate ideas to better support this client in day-to-day care. They added that they were very impressed with how the meeting with the staff stayed focused on the positives and was client-focused, while also ensuring staff safety.

Conclusion

Working with clients in a healthcare setting is usually very rewarding, but can at times be frustrating when they refuse to participate in necessary treatments. When a situation like this occurs, clients are often referred to as "challenging." Such frustration can be a byproduct of the interventions a clinician usually finds effective in situations like this not being effective and in fact at times this makes the situation with the client even worse; that is, the situation escalates. To find a more effective approach, the CBS program was developed as a way of seeking collaboration rather than compliance. The program is based on the already established Humanistic, Solution-Focused Coaching approach, as well as the Funnel of Optimal Functioning. Trained CBS coaches consult with staff who are stuck in their work with a challenging client. The CBS coaches work to collaborate with staff in a way that helps the staff be more collaborative with the client. We have found the CBS program to work and as the solution-focused approach advocates, "if it works do more of it," which we intend to do.

References

Baldwin, P., King, G., Evans, J., McDougall, S., Tucker, M.A., & Servais, M. (2013). Solution-focused coaching in pediatric rehabilitation: An integrated model for practice. *Physical & Occupational Therapy in Pediatrics, 33*(4), 467–483.

Cook, E. (2022). The funnel of optimal functioning: A model coach education. *The Coaching Psychologist, 18*, 43–58.

Law, M., Rosenbaum, P., King, G., Burke-Gaffney, J., Moning-Szkut, T., Kertoy, M., & Teplicky, R. (2003). Family-centred service sheets: 18 educational materials designed for parents, service providers, and organizations. Hamilton, ON, Canada, McMaster University, CanChild Centre for Childhood Disability Research.

Schwellnus, H. & Carnahan, H. (2014). Peer-coaching with health care professionals: What is the current status of the literature and what are the key components necessary in peer-coaching? A scoping review. *Medical Teacher, 36*(1), 38–46.

7 A Humanistic, Solution-Focused Approach to Working with Older Adults

Countering the Stigma of Ageism

Jacqueline Carver and Gilbert J. Greene

The rate of the aging population is increasing. By the year 2050, the number of individuals who are 65 years of age and older will reach 1.5 billion (Lederman & Shefler, 2023). Furthermore, the global population that is 65 years of age and older will increase to 16% by the year 2025 (Lederman & Shefler, 2023). Aging involves various physical, psychological, and social changes. Getting older increases the occurrence of various health problems. Older adults are more likely to experience friends and family passing away which can result in feelings of grief and social isolation. Such changes can result in older people having mental health issues. The mental health issues of older adults often are underdiagnosed, untreated, and do not receive proper follow-up care. Older adults need to receive appropriate mental health services to maintain their quality of life, both physically and mentally (PAN Foundation, 2021).

Because the aging population is growing, there is a need for mental health services tailored to the older adult population. Yet, at the same time, there are inadequate mental health services specifically for older adults. There are not enough programs or mental health professionals specializing in working with older adults. When older adults do get referred for mental health services, they are more likely to be prescribed only psychotropic medication and not offered psychotherapy (Frost, Beattie, Bhanu, et al., 2019). In fact, it is not uncommon for older adults to be overmedicated on psychotropic medications (Safer, 2019).

One reason for the lack of such services is the effect of ageism on designing and providing mental health services to older adults. It has been found that policymakers and service providers see older adults as not being able to benefit from mental health services because of the challenges, both physically and mentally, that are often inherent in getting older. Such views lead to stereotyping and stigma (Kang & Kim, 2022; Ward, 1977). Given these challenges, how might these issues be successfully addressed? This chapter will discuss a treatment approach that is well-suited for older adults and describe a unique program developed to provide mental health services in a rural area to older adults which uses that approach.

Aging, Ageism, and Mental Health Treatment

One barrier to older adults receiving mental health treatment or experiencing positive outcomes while receiving mental health treatment is ageism. Ageism is

DOI: 10.4324/9781003414490-9

stereotyping and discriminating against individuals because of their age (APA, 2014, 2020; Butler, 1969). According to Lederman & Shefler (2023, p. 351) "ageism is manifested in treating older people, aging, and old age in a uniform way, neglecting the heterogeneous, diverse, complex, and multifaceted nature of these constructs." In mental health settings, older adults are often seen as having too many problems and deficits and being too rigid to benefit from psychotherapy (Lederman & Shefler, 2023). However, most older adults adapt well to aging and can maintain good cognitive and physical health (Weir, 2023). In addition, most older adults can benefit from psychotherapy for a wide range of problems as well as younger adults can (APA, 2014, 2020; Lederman & Shefler, 2023; Karel, 2012). Yet, older adults are less likely to be referred for mental health therapy services. Even when older adults are referred for mental health services, they are less likely to receive adequate treatment as most mental health clinicians have not been properly trained in the unique needs of older adults (Weir, 2023).

When beginning treatment, most clients are feeling "demoralized," that is, feeling hopeless and lacking a sense of personal agency (Frank & Frank, 1991). Thus, any type of treatment should increase client hope and sense of personal agency along with ameliorating their presenting problems and symptoms. How a clinician communicates with clients affects whether hope and personal agency are activated in clients. Such activation is not likely to occur if the clinician has ageist beliefs. A clinician with ageist beliefs will have problems seeing beyond the problems and deficits of older adults and overlook their existing strengths, resources, and competencies (Lederman & Shefler, 2023).

Treating the Whole Person and Person-Centered Care

When clinicians do consider older adults' strengths and competencies along with their problems and deficits, they are then treating the whole person (Cook, 2020; Remen, 2008). That is, they realize that there is more to the client as a person and their story than just aging, problems, and illness. In Whole Person Care (WPC), the clinician-client relationship is the most important element (Thomas, Mitchell, Rich & Best, 2018). WPC is consistent with humanism. In a humanistic WPC approach, the clinician – client relationship is collaborative, and the client is invited to be an active participant in their care. Humanism views people as capable, autonomous, and having the potential to create solutions to increase positivity in their lives (Seligman, 2006). Humanism also affirms and empowers individuals by giving them confidence to utilize their inner resources and strengths (Seligman, 2006).

Also consistent with humanistic WPC is *person-centered care*. Person-centered care has been influenced by person-centered therapy and its humanistic underpinnings (Naldemirci, Lydal, Britten, et al., 2018). Person-centered care is an evidence-based approach that views clients as partners when determining the course of treatment in healthcare. Person-centered care involves making decisions alongside the client based on the client's needs, values, and preferences (Kogan et al., 2016). Person-centered clinicians accept, respect, and value their clients (Seligman, 2006). Treating older adults with respect and dignity means seeing the individual as a person and not just as an age (Giosa et al., 2022). Clinicians who utilize a person-centered approach recognize that older adults have intrinsic abilities for achieving their goals.

When taking a person-centered approach, it is important to allow enough time for dialogue between the older adult client and the clinician to build a trusting relationship. Clinicians need to talk *with* older adults rather than talking *at* them. Older adults have identified the importance of two-way information sharing as essential when building a trusting relationship with the clinician (Giosa et al., 2022). Communicating this way helps clinicians to identify clients' preferences, beliefs, and values regarding care and to be more engaged in services, thus leading to a higher quality of care (Kogan et al., 2016). In addition, research indicates that direct providers who utilize person-centered care tend to be satisfied and happy with their jobs, leading to less turnover (Kogan et al., 2016).

Despite the documented benefits of person-centered care, it lacks specifics on how to best operationalize it in clinician-client interactions. An approach that is consistent with person-centered care and provides more specifics on how to best create and maintain an effective clinician-client relationship is the solution-focused (SF) approach.

The Solution-Focused Approach (SFA)

The SFA is person-centered and effective in activating clients' strengths and resources. This approach is widely used in therapy and coaching in general (Grant, 2013; Murphy, 2024) and in medical and behavioral health settings specifically (Greene, Kondrat, Lee, et al., 2006; Zhang, Franklin, Currin-McCulloch, et al., 2018). Though the solution-focused approach originated in psychotherapy, in essence it is a way of communicating across a wide range of settings and situations (Shennan, 2019).

The SFA focuses on what's right with people and the future rather than their deficits and their past; its focus is on identifying and amplifying clients' strengths and competencies rather than remediating their deficits. The emphasis is on engaging clients in talking about change, their future, and solutions rather than their problems, deficits, and the past. Of course, clients need to have the time to tell their story which includes their past and problems. How clinicians respond to clients in this process provides the building blocks for developing and maintaining a positive therapeutic alliance. Then when the clinician believes that the client has felt heard and validated, the clinician begins to ask specific types of questions unique to the solution-focused approach that help to identify and amplify the client's strengths and resources leading to clients making the changes they desire. Though these questions have been discussed elsewhere in this book, we will briefly present the questions and some examples here.

Exception question – "When are there times the problem doesn't occur or is just a little bit better?"

Questions for identifying past exceptions – "When was the last time you did not feel depressed and you felt like your old self?"

The miracle questions – See elsewhere in this book for an example of the miracle question.

Scaling questions – "On a scale of 10 to 0 with 0 the worst the problem could be and 10 is the problem is completely gone, where are you on that scale today? When you feel like our work together is successfully completed, where would you like to be on the 10 – 0 scale? When will you know you have moved up one point on the 10 – 0 scale from where you are now?"

Relationship questions – "Who will be the first person to notice that you have moved up one point on the 10 – 0 scale? What will they notice different about you that will tell them you have moved up one point on that scale?"

Coping questions – "You've been depressed a long time. How do you cope with depression? How do you keep going?"

Personal agency questions – "What did you do to get yourself to move up one point on the scale since last week?"

Over the years, the SFA has been successfully used with older adults and their families (Bonjean, 1989, 2003; Chapin, Nelson-Becker, MacMillan & Sellon, 2016; Dahl, Bathel, and Carreon, 2000; Ebrahimi & Abdi, 2023; Giosa, Byrne & Stolee, 2021; Ingersoll-Dayton & Berit, 1993; Ingersoll-Dayton, Schroepfer & Prynce, 1999; and Wang, Wang, Wang, et al., 2023) in addition it has been found to help in reducing stigma in clients with mental health issues (Ayar, Karasu & Sahpolat, 2021; Erdogan & Demir, 2022).

Stages Behavioral Health: A Solution-Focused Person-Centered Program

The Area Agency on Aging (AAA3) in Lima, Ohio saw a need for behavioral health programming within the agency to overcome barriers that older adults face when they are referred to community-based behavioral health services. For example, out-of-pocket expenses, the lack of available providers that meet credentialing requirements for Medicare, the lack of access to services in general, and the lack of transportation, especially in rural areas, are barriers that prevent older adults from receiving the necessary behavioral health services. Thus, Stages Behavioral Health Program (SBHP) was launched at AAA3 in 2021, which has a seven-county catchment area with a majority of the area served being rural. In Ohio, there are 12 Area Agencies on Aging and the Lima, Ohio AAA3 catchment area is the only one with an internal behavioral health program. The SBHP believes that services must be available and accessible to the older adult population and tailored to their needs. Thus, the SBHP provides services in the office, in long-term care facilities, in-home, and via telehealth.

Solution-Focused Person-Centered Care in Practice with Older Adults

In developing the SBHP, the first author of this chapter (JC) saw that it was essential to administer the program in a way that allowed older adults to feel accepted and not judged, and to allow clients to maintain control and autonomy when receiving services. It was clear that there was a significant need for a person-centered and strength-based behavioral health program tailored to the older adult population. Therefore, to create such a program, the clinician understood the importance of working collaboratively with clients to identify and understand their values and beliefs.

In addition to collaborating with the client, the SFA views the client as the expert in all facets of their lives. For instance, clinicians will take a "one down" position within the therapeutic relationship, which allows the client to lead the sessions as the clinician leads from "one step behind" during the therapeutic process. It is essential to understand what the client wants to accomplish when they decide to pursue behavioral health services. Therefore, the SBHP clinician begins each meeting by asking the client something like "what are your best hopes for what you want to accomplish in the time we have together?" At the end of every session, the clinician asks the client if he or she would like to reschedule and, if so, when would the client like to return. This is one way to allow the client to be the expert, guide the therapeutic process, and contribute to a sense of autonomy, control, and personal agency.

The SFA encourages the client to identify, use, and build upon their prior solutions. The clinician must engage in active listening, thereby using the client's language, which promotes a focus on the client identifying solutions and strengths (Jerome et al., 2023). For instance, when a client of the SBHP identified that she wanted to feel "in control," instead of the clinician assuming she knew what the client meant by "control," she asked the client to give her definition of control and what it looks like for the client to have control in her environment. When the clinician follows what works best for the client and utilizes the client's language, this leads to collaboration between the clinician and the client. Also, the client is more likely to formulate solutions when the clinician utilizes the client's language (Jerome et al., 2023).

Exception Questions

A female client in her early 60s, "Bev," requested behavioral health therapy and stated that the presenting problem was waking up in the morning feeling intense panic that led to ongoing anxiety throughout the rest of the day. The client stated she had no idea what was contributing to the panic and that she had been unsuccessful at trying to reduce the symptoms. After hearing the client's explanation of the problem, validating the frustration that she was experiencing, and reflecting in order to build rapport, the clinician encouraged the client to identify an exception to the problem:

Bev: I wake up in the morning in a panic and then I feel anxious for the rest of the day.

Clinician: When has there been a time that you woke up in the morning and the panic was less intense or not present at all?

Bev:	Actually, a couple of weeks ago I woke up, I felt refreshed, and I didn't feel panicked or anxious.
Clinician:	What was different about that morning?
Bev:	The night before I went to bed knowing that I was going to wake up and work in the yard and then pick up my grandkids. I had plans to take the grandkids to a movie and then out to eat.
Clinician:	It sounds like having a plan for the next day had a positive impact on how you woke up that morning.
Bev:	It did. And now that I think about it, on the days that I work I don't wake up in a panic. It's only on the days that I don't have a plan or project to work on.

By exploring exceptions to when the problem is present, the client was able to identify that having a plan for the next day negates the panic and anxiety that she has experienced in the mornings. The client then decided to do an experiment that included making a weekly schedule of activities that she wanted to accomplish during each day. The client discovered that adhering to the schedule led to waking up without panicking and in fact, the client stated she woke up feeling a sense of motivation.

Questions for Identifying Past Exceptions

"Adam," a male client in his 70s who was self-referred, indicated that he had been feeling depressed and hopeless. Adam explained he had retired two years ago and felt "useless" ever since. Adam explained that he used to volunteer as well and that he is no longer doing that. Adam stated he had pain in his knees and was no longer able to engage in activities that he used to engage in, such as repairing his home and woodcarving. Adam continued to write, which was another activity that he enjoyed, yet stated he did not feel motivated to write like he had in the past. Adam could not identify any current or recent exceptions so the clinician asked him about past exceptions:

Adam:	I'm just so down. I used to be so active and now that I have this pain, I just sit at home. My wife and I used to travel, I used to volunteer and write, and now I just sit. My mind doesn't feel old, but my body does. I'm turning into one of those grumpy old men that just sits in a chair all day not doing anything. I can't even fix things in my own house. Getting old is depressing.
Clinician:	When was the last time you didn't feel that depression?
Adam:	I'd say a couple years ago when I was still working and volunteering. I was also writing and giving talks in the community. I went to several businesses and gave talks about finances. That's what my books are about.
Clinician:	It sounds like sharing your knowledge with others is important to you.
Adam:	It is, I was useful, I had a purpose, I was happy.

In this example, Adam was able to identify that he did not feel depressed when he was sharing his knowledge with others through work and volunteering in the community. With further exception questions and future-oriented questions, Adam was able to identify how he could continue to contribute to the community. Adam started by mentoring a young businessman in the community and eventually started writing consistently again. By the sixth session, Adam stated he was no longer experiencing symptoms of depression, he felt hopeful, and he stated he felt a sense of purpose again. Also, once Adam began mentoring and writing again, he reported that the pain in his knees was less intense.

Along with identifying past exceptions, this example also demonstrates how one may experience the stigma of internalized ageism. Adam identified himself as a "grumpy old man" who "just sits," which is a common stereotype that depicts older adults as inactive and unproductive individuals. By taking a solution-focused approach, the clinician was able to view the client as a person who has strengths and competencies instead of an older adult who was experiencing physical pain that led to a sedentary lifestyle. In addition, the solution-focused approach not only led Adam to focus on his strengths, but it also aided the clinician in focusing on the whole person who is resilient instead of focusing on any ageist beliefs she may have had. As a result, the clinician viewed Adam as a person, not an age, and did not focus on perceived age-related deficits yet focused on Adam's ability to make positive change leading to a positive outlook for his future.

The Scaling Question

The scaling question is a way for the client to quantify their current and desired future situations along a scale ranging from 10 to 0. This allows the clinician to collaboratively develop a treatment plan with the client using the client's language and frame-of-reference. It can also assist clients in recognizing progress that they made from session to session.

A male client in his 70s, who will be referred to as "Stan," attended his first session with the clinician, stating that he felt depressed and was isolating from others. The client stated that he stayed in his house all day and night and had no desire to know what was taking place outside of his home. The client was retired and lived alone and reported a history of having close friendships, yet stated he no longer had a desire to interact with his friends. The client referred to the depression as the "heavy darkness." Below is an example of how the clinician utilized scaling questions along with utilizing the client's language.

Clinician: On a scale of 10 to 0 with 0 being the heaviest the darkness could be and 10 being the heavy darkness is completely gone, where are you on that scale today?

Stan: It's a 1, the heavy darkness is always there.

Clinician: When you know that we have successfully completed our work together, where will you be on the 10–0 scale?

Stan:	It will be at 7. I don't think it will get to a 10 just because life happens and so many of my friends are gone now, but I think I can get to a 7.
Clinician:	When will you know that you have moved up one point on the scale from where you are today?
Stan:	I will open my curtains and actually let the sunlight in.

The Relationship Question

Continuing with Stan, the clinician asked him the relationship question to help to interpersonally contextualize his desired change.

Clinician:	And who will be the first person, a person that you have in your life, who will notice that you have moved up one point on this scale?
Stan:	It will be my friend Max. He's known me for years, ever since we were kids, and he knows that I'm not myself. He knows that I'm depressed.
Clinician:	What will Max notice is different about you when you move up one point on the 10–0 scale?
Stan:	He'll notice because I won't be so stuck in that darkness. He'll drive by my house and see some action. I won't be so closed in.
Clinician:	What else will Max notice?
Stan:	He'll probably notice that I'm going outside again and keeping up with my yard and landscaping like I used to.

The Miracle Question

To assist clients in formulating goals, the SBHP clinician uses the "miracle question" to assist clients in identifying and describing what will be different when the presenting problem is no longer a problem. This description of what will be different also identifies behavioral indicators that specify not only what clients will notice has changed, but also what their family and other supportive people in their lives will notice has changed (the relationship question).

For example, "Sara," responded to the miracle question and identified changes that will indicate the problem is no longer a problem when the goal has been completed. Sara further narrowed this down by identifying the very first step towards completing this goal. Upon reviewing the treatment plan, which was developed collaboratively with Sara using Sara's words and frame-of-reference, Sara replied to the clinician with, "Wow, you really listened to me." This is why it is imperative that the clinician works to understand the problem and goal from the client's point of view with little interpretation and analysis by the clinician. The client identifies the goals without the clinician making assumptions about what may be at the root of the presenting issue (Jerome et al., 2023). Furthermore, identified goals should be obtainable for the client to continue to move forward and progress (Jerome et al., 2023). For example, Sara referred to her goal and the very first step in sessions and identified when she had completed the very first step.

The Coping Question

Coping questions are useful when the client is unable to identify any exceptions to the problem. In the case here, the clinician continued to use Stan's language when asking a coping question.

Clinician: I can see that the darkness is feeling heavy. How do you cope with the heavy darkness?

Stan: My cat. I got my cat and it's my responsibility to take care of him. It wouldn't be right if I didn't. I care about my cat. I care about my friends.

Clinician: I can hear that despite the heavy darkness, you continue to care about others, and you continue to be responsible.

Stan: That's just part of who I am. I care and I take responsibility.

In this case example, Stan was able to identify strengths that he has and how he continues to utilize these strengths, caring for others, caring for his cat, and being a responsible individual.

Personal Agency Question

Personal agency questions help to activate and strengthen the client's sense of agency.

When Stan returned for a session one week later, he identified progress that he had made using the 10 to 0 scale.

Clinician: I'm wondering where you are on the 10–0 scale today, with 0 being the heaviest the darkness could be and 10 being the heavy darkness is no longer present.

Stan: I would say I'm at a 2 this week.

Clinician: What did you do to move up on the scale since last week?

Stan: I opened my curtains. I closed them again in the evening, but I did open them during the day and let the sunlight in. I knew my cat would like looking out the window too.

Stan was able to identify how he moved up one point and he also recognized that his pet cat, who he continued to take care of, was a source of motivation to open his curtains but ultimately Stan motivated himself to take the necessary action. Even though the heavy darkness was still present, Stan was able to positively change his behavior indicating a sense of personal agency.

The End of Session Note

To make the session even more individualized, as the clinician actively listens to Gwen during sessions, the clinician will make a "note" that includes strengths that Gwen has identified during the session, using Gwen's own words and frame-of-reference. This "note" serves as a reminder to Gwen regarding her strengths and is something Gwen can refer to between sessions. The note usually consists of bullet points highlighting strengths Gwen has identified, which may include writing down words or phrases that Gwen said during the session, such as "I like to laugh," "I was determined," and/or "I talked about it and that helped." If the clinician had focused on the negative changes Gwen is experiencing due to dementia versus the strengths and resilience that Gwen continues to utilize, Gwen may have discontinued services as the therapy sessions would have not been any different from the deficit-based medical models that she indicated she is "tired of."

Conclusion

The rate of the older adult population is increasing, yet accessible mental health services are not increasing. There is both a need for increased access to mental health services and increased quality mental health services that are tailored to the needs of older adults. Further research is needed to address what therapeutic processes best address the needs of the older adult population. Also, further education is needed to reduce the effects of ageism and its effects on mental health. For instance, training mental health clinicians in solution-focused therapy may be more effective and efficient in ameliorating clinicians' ageist beliefs. If clinicians are trained in the SFA, then they will be focused on the strengths and abilities of the older adult client, not their deficits, shifting one's perception of aging from a negative view to a positive one thus reducing stigma.

After hearing their stories, it is clear that older adults want the opportunity to be an active participant in their mental and physical health needs. Encouraging clients to identify existing strengths promotes resilience, agency, and hope, leading clients to see that they already have strengths and resources, thereby increasing their confidence and optimism regarding change and finding solutions (Jerome et al., 2023). Both person-centered and solution-focused approaches allow the client and the clinician to collaborate so that the client is heard, respected, and validated instead of stigmatized. Taking a nonjudgmental and strength-based approach whereby the client's strengths and successes are highlighted is vital. It is time that we appreciate and acknowledge older adults as the experts on their needs and wants throughout older adulthood.

References

American Psychological Association. (2012). Guidelines for psychological practice with older adults. *American Psychologist, 69*(1), 34–65.
American Psychological Association (2020). APA Resolution on Ageism. Available at: https://www.apa.org/about/policy/resolution-ageism.pdf
Ayar, D., Karasu, F., & Sahpolat, M. (2021). The relationship between levels of solution-focused thinking and internalized stigma and social functionality in mental disorders. *Perspectives in Psychiatric Care, 58*(4), 1399–1409.
Bonjean, M.J. (1989). Solution-focused psychotherapy with families caring for an Alzheimer's patient. *Journal of Psychotherapy & the Family, 5*(1–2), 197–210.

Bonjean, M.J. (2003). Solution-focused therapy: Elders enhancing exceptions. In J. Ronch & J. A. Goldfrield (eds), *Mental Wellness in Aging: Strengths-Based Approaches* (pp. 201–235). Health Professions Press.

Butler, R.N. (1969). Ageism: Another form of bigotry. *The Gerontologist, 9*(4), 243–246.

Chapin, R., Nelson-Becker, N., MacMillan, K., & Sellon, A. (2016). Strengths-based and solution-focused practice with older adults: New applications. In: D. B. Kaplan & B. Berkman (eds), *The Oxford Handbook of Social Work in Health and Aging* (2nd ed., pp. 63–71). Oxford University Press.

Cook, E. (2022). The funnel of optimal functioning: A model for coach education. *The Coaching Psychologist, 18*(2), 43–58.

Dahl, R., Bathel, D., & Carreon, C. (2000). The use of solution-focused therapy with an elderly population. *Journal of Systemic Therapies, 19*(4), 45–55.

Ebrahimi, P. & Abdi, M. (2023). The effectiveness of solution-focused approach on increasing social adjustment and reducing clinical depression in elderly women of Kermanshah. *Aging Psychology, 9*(2), 151–165.

Erdogan, E. & Demir, S. (2022). The effect of solution focused group psychoeducation applied to schizophrenia patients on self-esteem, perception of subjective recovery and internalized stigmatization. *Issues in Mental Health Nursing, 43*(10), 944–954.

Frank, J. D. & Frank, J. B. (1991). *Persuasion & Healing: A Comparative Study of Psychotherapy*. Johns Hopkins University Press.

Frost, R., Beattie, A., Bhanu, C., Walters, K., & Ben-Shlomo, Y. (2019). Management of depression and referral of older people to psychological therapies: A systematic review of qualitative studies. *British Journal of General Practice, 69*(680), e171–e181.

Giosa, J. L., Byrne, K., & Stolee, P. (2021). Person- and family-centred goal-setting for older adults in Canadian home care: A solution-focused approach. *Health & Social Care in the Community, 30*(5), e2445–e2456.

Grant, A.M. (2013). Steps to solutions: A process for putting solution-focused coaching principles into practice. *The Coaching Psychologist, 9*(1), 36–44.

Greene, G. J., Kondrat, D. C., Lee, M. Y., Clement, J., Siebert, H., Meritzer, R. A. et al. (2006). A solution-focused approach to case management and recovery with consumers who have a severe mental disability. *Families in Society, 87*(3), 339–350.

Ingersoll-Dayton, B. & Rader, J. (1993). Searching for solutions: Mental health consultation in nursing homes. *Clinical Gerontologist, 13*(1), 33–50.

Ingersoll-Dayton, B., Schroepfer, T., & Pryce, J. (1999). The effectiveness of a solution-focused approach for problem behaviors among nursing home residents. *Journal of Gerontological Social Work, 32*(3), 49–64.

Jerome, L., McNamee, P., Abdel-Halim, N., Elliot, K., & Woods, J. (2023). Solution-focused approaches in adult mental health research: A conceptual literature review and narrative synthesis. *Frontiers in Psychiatry, 14*, 1–15.

Kang, H. & Kim, H. (2022). Ageism and psychological well-being among older adults: A systematic review. *Gerontology & Geriatric Medicine, 8*(1), 1–22.

Kogan, A. C., Wilber, K., & Mosqueda, L. (2016). Moving toward implementation of person-centered care for older adults in community-based medical and social service settings: 'You only get things done when working in concert with clients'. *Journal of American Geriatric Society, 64*(1), e8–e14.

Lederman, S. & Shefler, G. (2023). Psychotherapy with older adults: Ageism and the therapeutic process. *Psychotherapy Research, 33*(3), 350–361.

Murphy, J. J. (2024). *Solution-Focused Therapy*. American Psychological Association.

Naldemirci, O., Lydahl, D., Britten, N., Elam, M., Moore, L., & Wolf, A. (2018). Tenacious assumptions of person-centred care? Exploring tensions and variations in practice. *Health: An Interdisciplinary Journal for the Study of Health, Illness & Medicine, 22*(1), 54–71.

PAN Foundation. (2021). Addressing gaps in mental health services for older adults. *Issue Brief*, 1–14.

Petrova, N. N. & Khvostikova, D. A. (2021). Prevalence, structure, and risk factors for mental disorders in older people. *Advances in Gerontology, 11*(4), 409–415.

Remen, R. N. (2008). Practicing a medicine of the whole person: An opportunity for healing. *Hematology/Oncology Clinics of North America, 22*(4), 767–773.

Safer, D. J. (2019). Overprescribed medications for US adults: Four major examples. *Journal of Clinical Medicine Research, 11*(9), 617–622.

Seligman, L. (2006). *Theories of Counseling and Psychotherapy* (2nd ed.). Pearson Education.

Shennan, G. (2019). *Solution-Focused Practice: Effective Communication to Facilitate Change*. Red Globe Press.

Thomas, H., Mitchell, G., Rich, J., & Best, M. (2018). Definition of whole person care in general practice in the English language literature: A systematic review. *BMJ Open, 8*(12), 1–12.

Wang, C., Wang, C., Wang, J., Yu, N. X., Tang, Y., Liu, Z. et al. (2023). Effectiveness of solution-focused group counseling on depression and cognition among Chinese older adults: A cluster randomized controlled trial. *Research on Social Work Practice, 33*(5), 530–543.

Ward, R. A. (1977). The impact of subjective age and stigma on older persons. *Journal of Gerontology, 32*(2), 227–232.

Weir, K. (2023). Ageism is one of the last socially acceptable prejudices. Psychologists are working to change that. *American Psychological Association, 54*(2), 36–48.

Zhang, A., Franklin, C., Currin-McCulloch, J., Park, S., & Kim, J. (2018). The effectiveness of strengths-based, solution-focused brief therapy in medical settings: A systematic review and meta-analysis of randomized controlled trials. *Journal of Behavioral Medicine, 41*(2), 139–151.

8 Humanistic, Solution-Focused Nursing in the Paediatric Psychopharmacology Clinic

An Antidote to Burnout

Cathy Petta

Nurses deal with client problems – a lot of problems! These problems can be physical, mental, or both. It is no secret that nurses not only deal with a lot of problems, but they see many clients with problems every day, day in and day out. These demands of the job can lead to nurses experiencing burnout (Ge et al., 2022) and job turnover (Leiter & Maslach, 2009). When someone feels burned out, they may experience exhaustion, emotional depletion, depersonalization, and detachment from clients and the job, cynicism, pessimism, hopelessness, lacking job-related personal accomplishment and efficacy, and so on. Burnout not only negatively affects nurses, but also the quality of client care suffers (Theofanidis et al., 2022). An approach that has been found to help with burnout is solution-focused coaching and counselling (SFC; Luo et al., 2019; Medina & Beyebach, 2014). The solution-focused approach assumes that all people have strengths, competencies, and resources that can be utilized in achieving their goals. It has been found that the SF approach can increase positive emotions (Kim & Franklin, 2015), hope (Kim et al., 2022), and self-efficacy (Akgul-Gundogdu & Selcuk-Tosun, 2021) in addition to preventing or reducing burnout. In this chapter, I will describe my experience with burnout and journey of learning and using a Humanistic, Solution-Focused Approach for successfully dealing with it in my job as a nurse in a paediatric psychopharmacology clinic.

My Burnout Experience

Currently, I work as a registered nurse (RN) in the Psychopharmacology Clinic at Holland Bloorview Kids Rehabilitation Hospital. Kids who are referred to the clinic must have a diagnosis of autism and/or intellectual disability (ID) and/or a genetic syndrome associated with autism or ID. They also must have tried and "failed" at using at least one medication targeting the behaviour of concern. What this means in practice is that the families and children who come to our clinic are generally in crisis in terms of being able to safely support their children at home, at school, and in the community. My role in the clinic is to follow up with families and community agencies/services/schools, etc. on clinic recommendations, including medication monitoring (effectiveness and side effects), behaviour interventions, and community supports and service. In practice, this means having telephone conversations with families, schools, community agencies and services,

DOI: 10.4324/9781003414490-10

child protection services, and group home staff, mostly about how the child is struggling to be successful because of behaviours which negatively impact how they interact with the people in their life and their environment.

I started my nursing career over 30 years ago in North Wales as a hospital-trained Registered Nurse. I had completed a bachelor's degree in an unrelated field (Environmental Studies), returned to my hometown, and found jobs in my field of study to be non-existent. Contemplating my options, I landed on nursing as a career path; I wanted to be of service and "help" people – my exact words during my nursing school interview. I have continued in this vein of wanting to help people for the last 30 years. Early on in my career, helping people and being of service became operationalized in my mind as it being my responsibility to figure out what was wrong with my patient to be able to fix and make everything better for them. I eventually discovered doing this to be a path to burnout.

I am a nurse nearing the end of my career, being over 60 years old. Five years ago, I was considering my options for early retirement or possible career change. Despite having excellent self-care habits and a life outside of work, my energy and enthusiasm for my job was very low. I was distancing myself from my job and was negative and cynical when it came to thinking about my work, and I was questioning my ability to continue to provide adequate, never mind excellent, nursing care for the families and kids of my clinic. In short, I was experiencing burnout. Fortunately, learning about and integrating a humanistic, solution-focused approach to my interactions with the clients and families of my clinic has been instrumental in countering burnout and extending my nursing career.

Person-/Patient-Centred Care and the Humanistic, Solution-Focused Approach

The hospital I work at has been a leader in embedding the concepts and principals of Patient- and Family-Centred Care (PFCC) – the belief that clients and families are an equal partner in their healthcare journey (Johnson et al., 2008). The four core principles of PFCC are dignity and respect, information-sharing, participation, and collaboration. I have always understood the principles of client and family care on the macro level, and despite wanting to practise in a client- and family-centred way, I was not clear on how to bring this approach into my everyday practice. The Humanistic, Solution-Focused (HSF) approach has provided me with a highly pragmatic framework and tools to operationalize the idea that clients and families are authors of their own healthcare journey (McPherson et al., 2019).

The SF approach has also relieved me of the burden to fix and make everything better for people while not relieving me of the responsibility of doing my job within my scope of practice. By bringing the humanistic, SF approach to my practice, I have been enabled to interact with my clients and families in a way that consistently *elicits, amplifies, and reinforces* their strengths and resources (Macdonald, 2007), facilitating them to work towards their own preferred future as articulated by them. Ultimately, clients are the authors and authority of their own healthcare journey (McPherson et al., 2019).

My Humanistic, Solution-Focused Journey

The Hook

My solution-focused journey began about 6 years ago when my hospital trained all clinicians (in the form of a two-day workshop) in solution-focused coaching. I remember that first two-day workshop as being interesting and exciting; in a brief 20-minute solution-focused practice conversation with a colleague, I was able to facilitate my partner devising a solution to a problem which had plagued her for many years. Despite the elation I felt with this small success using this novel (to me) approach, I still didn't really understand how this approach could transform my practice.

Following that initial SF training, I was awarded some funds to attend a work-related conference or workshop. This solution-focused conference actually transformed my experience of my work – I am not exaggerating. I was so excited by every presentation and was starting to envision how the approach could be applicable to my practice. Not many presentations related to healthcare; however, the last talk was from a social worker working in child protection, who opened her talk by saying that she had been burnt out, and had dreaded answering the phone and people calling expecting her to give answers and solutions to their problems which she didn't have. The burden of responsibility of trying to meet those demands was wearing her down and making her want to quit. She then said that *she no longer dreads answering the phone!* **That was the hook. That was me.** I dreaded answering the phone; I felt hopeless, useless, and so burdened by the responsibility to fix the unfixable. I realized that I couldn't continue doing things the way I had been doing them for so many years – look for the problem, come up with solutions, and convince families to follow through within the constraints of a less-than-perfect healthcare system. This moment was the start of my journey in humanistic, solution-focused nursing practice. When I got back to work the following week, I heard that Dr Elaine Cook had been hired to continue the process of embedding the solution-focused approach to care at our hospital; I sought her out and my journey began.

Certified Solution-Focused Healthcare Coach and Facilitator Training

Elaine invited me to be in one of the first cohorts to go through the certified solution-focused healthcare coach and facilitator program, the program she developed, the first of its kind; solution-focused coaching in a healthcare setting. For me, this program operationalized our hospital's mandate to provide client- and family-centred care, equal partnership between client and family and clinician, in a way I could bring into my practice even a little at a time. Research at our hospital investigating the SF approach and its impact on families and clinicians has demonstrated positive outcomes for both (King et al., 2019; King et al., 2022). As previously mentioned, I had attended a two-day workshop on the SF approach at the hospital and had a tantalizing glimpse of how this approach could transform how I felt about my practice and the impact on my interactions with clients and families.

However, until I embarked on the certification process, I was not able to sustain using the approach on a day-to-day level in my practice.

The certification program had two elements: formal, didactic learning on the elements of the approach; and informal or peer coaching sessions where we practised our learning and coaching in real coaching situations with our peers. Practising our newly emerging coaching skills in a safe, non-judgemental environment supervised by an experienced coach was transformative. I was able to take what I was learning and practising into my clinical conversations with clients and families of the clinic. A little at a time. My default of believing it was my responsibility to do what needed to be done to fix my clients and families was and is hard-wired. This ingrained belief that I was responsible for my clients' and families' health and well-being was my default approach to nursing practice.

I was nearing retirement age (well considering early retirement at 58 anyway!) at the time I embarked on this humanistic, solution-focused journey. Despite always having enjoyed my job, being considered a valuable team member, and always receiving excellent feedback about my abilities from colleagues and clients, I was dreading going to work, dreading that phone ringing, worried constantly about the kids in our clinic and their families, and worried about my perceived hopelessness of their situation and my helplessness to help them. Despite all this, I was always impressed by the families' tenacity, resilience, ability to show up every day in every situation for their kids; to advocate for them at school, in social and family situations, to endure endless waiting lists for services and support which didn't always deliver what was hoped for, to keep showing up no matter how they felt, trying to ensure their kids were able to live the best life possible. Many of the families were despairing, many with mental health issues themselves, isolated from community and family because of the challenges others have supporting and interacting successfully with autistic kids and youth, many with English as a second language trying to navigate a system which is hard enough for native language speakers to access and understand. And, yet, here they were all coming to appointments, calling asking for help, time and time and time again. I could see what incredible strength and resilience these people had and yet before SF came into my practice I could not envision and enact how to support families in harnessing those strengths and resources already being utilized, maybe subconsciously, and apply those same strengths and resources to the problems they were encountering daily.

What I also failed to see at this point was my own ability to keep showing up, despite feelings of hopelessness and helplessness about my ability to help. My expert knowledge and experience in the area I work in, my innate ability to connect with people in a way they seem to feel is a genuine interest in their well-being, my willingness to keep answering that phone, to keep showing up for them, to advocate on their behalf, to keep trying to connect them with resources and support, to keep listening to their need to talk about the problems and seemingly insurmountable issues they face every day, to keep trying to figure out what it is they need and to help them get it, to keep showing up despite how I felt.

For the last couple of years, I was beginning to only see my failure to fix everything and neglected to notice what I was actually doing, the inherent strengths and resources I was bringing to every conversation I had. I had forgotten my own wholeness (Remen, 1998, 2008). I believed I had been broken by the system I worked in. This approach offered me a route back to remembering my wholeness. A route to relieve me of the crushing responsibility I felt for everyone's well-being, not by abandoning them and leaving them to fend for themselves, but by offering a means to facilitate them, noticing, remembering, and accessing their own wholeness, strengths, and resources (inner and outer) so they can truly be the authors of their own healthcare journey (Remen, 1998, 2008).

A Little at a Time: Using the Scaling Question

One of the first things I was coached on during the program peer coaching session was how I can apply all the coaching skills and SF knowledge to my practice and conversations I have on a daily basis with clients and families of my clinic. My peer coaches started off the conversation in the usual manner by a contracting question: How will you know this conversation has been useful for you? I wanted to be able to embed the SF approach in my nursing practice. The coaches proceeded to explore what difference embedding the approach would make for me, who would notice, what I would notice – these were some of the questions asked. They then asked me a *scaling question* – on a scale of 10–0, where 10 is exactly where I want to be and 0 is not that, where am I? I was fairly low on the scale, around a 3, and I was a 3 not a 2 because I was learning more and more about SF because of my participation in the program, I had a desire to start embedding the approach more, and I was trying out some of the questions, mainly the "best hopes" question at the beginning of clinic visits or phone calls with families and kids. They also explored what I might be doing differently at a 3.5 that I am not already doing at a 3. This permission to start embedding the approach in small steps was transformational for me: it helped me focus on building on what I was already doing rather than what I am not doing. One of the first strategies I decided to start practising was holding the basic premise that everyone has *inherent strengths and resources* despite how things may seem or sound; that everyone is *whole at their core* and bringing this core belief into every interaction I had with families. I would then begin to notice what difference holding this belief made to the conversations I was having with families. I think the difference it made is best illustrated by an example of a real conversation I had not long after this coaching session.

A Case Example of Strengths, Resources, and Wholeness

I had a call from one of our clinic parents, a mother of an autistic girl who had extreme challenges with ADHD symptoms – unable to focus or stay still for more than a few seconds, as well as being very impulsive, which could lead to safety issues. The child had also experienced severe emotional trauma and physical abuse in her young life. Mum had also experienced abuse in intimate relationships. Mum had had her other children apprehended by child protection services in the past, as well as having a history of mental health issues. Mum could appear to be very combative and aggressive in her verbal interactions with the clinic team when she was experiencing challenges in supporting her child's behaviour. On the face of it, this mum seemed broken by what life had thrown at her. When I started holding this *core belief of her wholeness*, I was able to see her in a different light. I saw how much she loved this child and how she had fought to keep her despite constant child protection involvement. I saw how she showed up for every appointment despite living an hour-and-a-half away from our hospital. I noticed that she had a very close relationship with her daughter despite all the arguing and challenges. I noticed how resourceful she was at accessing community supports and services for herself and her child. I saw how relentlessly she advocated for her child at the school, attempting to get her child the best placement in the school system possible. In fact, once I started noticing this mum's strengths and resources, *I could not not see them anymore.* This mum did not see herself as whole, though. She would call with a list of problems and issues that she wanted us to fix for her and could get quite annoyed when we were unable to make everything better. She would not remember the progress her daughter had made over the years and her part in bringing it about. She wanted something done about every perceived crisis situation immediately.

She called this one day very escalated about a situation at home where the child (who was a pre-teen by now) was being extremely combative and arguing constantly with her mum about everything mum wanted her to do. Mum was demanding that we make medication changes to address this behaviour as she couldn't cope. Her voice was loud and angry and I could sense her level of agitation even though this was a phone call, not an in-person visit. We had already spoken to mum at the last clinic visit about how this behaviour was not able to be addressed with medication, that it was a normal part of development, and the child needed to learn. However, this was not the time to remind mum of this – she was very low on the Funnel of Optimal Functioning (FOF; Cook, 2022) and would not have been able to process this information in a way that would have been helpful for her. Instead, I listened to her, breathed slowly and deeply to keep myself calm, acknowledged what she was saying with calm, quiet expressions of "Ok," "right," "yes," and all the time listening for her wholeness and strengths and resources despite the problem talk. Eventually (and it probably didn't take more than 5 minutes), she calmed down enough that I was able to be curious about what she was already doing. I remembered the close relationship she had with her daughter and how much she loved her.

Asking the Exception Question

I asked her to tell me about a time in the last week when she and her daughter had spent some time – even if it was only just a few moments – doing something together that they both had enjoyed. Mum didn't even skip a beat – in fact, she seemed a little offended that I assumed they had only spent a little time in the week doing things they both enjoyed. She told me about the time they had spent making a little garden in their tiny backyard out of planters, how the both of them had hauled back the soil from Walmart and planted seeds and watered them and were looking forward to watching them grow. I tentatively asked whether there was anything else they had done and she proceeded to tell me about the times they spend reading together, and mum reminded me that reading is one of the child's favourite things to do. In fact, mum said she would really love the teachers to send her a reading list for her child to choose books from the library as the child reads so much she gets through her reading homework so fast. By asking mum about *exceptions* in the recent past where she and her daughter had been able to get along and enjoy each other's company, she was able to move up the FOF to a place where she was able to see other possibilities other than staying in a place where she felt frustrated and angry at our inability to fix the problem of her daughter being so oppositional. At the end of the phone call, she had made a plan to talk to the school about additional reading resources for her daughter.

Applying the Funnel of Optimal Functioning

The funnel of optimal functioning (Cook, 2022) has proved to be one of the most useful tools and concepts for me to use in all my interactions – with families, kids, colleagues, and even personal relationships outside of work. When the person I am talking with is low on the funnel as evidenced by tone and cadence of voice, emotional escalation, and other visual and auditory cues, I am able to match my response to where they are. For example, in the conversation above, I knew the mum was low down in the funnel – yelling loudly, fast cadence of talk, repeating over and over that she can't cope and needs the doctor to prescribe more medication. This tells me she is unable to process more information (questioning, suggestions, etc.) and I need to hold space for her – give her time to talk uninterrupted, model deep breathing and slow, calm speech when I do talk, acknowledge quietly what she is saying and not ask questions about why she is feeling the way she is feeling, and reflecting back what she is saying in her own words with no judgement or suggestions. I am also mentally taking note of her strengths and resources as she is talking. When I noticed that she was calming down, I was able to acknowledge what she has said and how difficult things have been and then ask questions about possibilities leading with constraints, namely, "despite things being so difficult how are you managing?", and then when I perceive that mum is ready to do some more advanced cognitive processing and self-reflection – as she starts to move higher up the funnel, I asked her the *exception question*: "Think about a time in the last week or so when you and R were not arguing, when you were enjoying each other's company, even for a short time; what was different about that time?" These questions help mum to become aware of what she already has been doing to manage the situation and even remember there are times when the problem is not so intense – nothing is a problem 100% of the time at 100% frequency and 100% intensity (Macdonald, 2007). These questions serve to continue to move mum higher up the funnel and access those higher centres of cognitive functioning and well-being. As a result, she was able to think about what a next step may be to help her daughter and herself based on what she identifies as their strengths – getting access to more books that they can read together.

Using the Scaling Question: A Case Example

My favourite solution-focused strategy is the use of scaling questions. I received a phone call from the mother of one of our clinic kids, a 9-year-old boy with autism and ADHD. We had started him on a small dose of a medication at the clinic visit a few weeks prior to her call and she was calling to give an update. I was still fairly new in the SF program and not very confident about asking SF questions and did not start off with a "what's better" question. I asked the usual "how are things go-ing" and mum launched into a description of how bad things were – he was "never" doing his homework without a fight, he couldn't focus for more than a few seconds, he argued constantly with parents about every little thing they asked of him, he "never" listened, etc. It seemed to go on and on and not one positive thing was mentioned by mum. Once she stopped giving me the list of problems that needed to be fixed by us, I knew that I had to acknowledge where she was in terms of how difficult she was finding things, as well as starting to explore with her what might be working even just a little despite all the challenges she and her son were experi-encing. I asked her a *scaling question* based on the information she had given me.

Scaling questions in solution-focused work score from high to low, that is, 10 is the best-case scenario and 0 is not that. This is a different approach from our usual medical scales such as the pain scale, where 10 is the worse pain and 0 is the absence of pain. I asked mum on a scale of 10 to 0 where 10 is the most satisfied she is with her son's behavior and 0 was not that, where is she? Given that her list of problems was quite extensive, I assumed she would be pretty low on the scale; however, she told me she was about a 7!!! I went on to explore what was different for her at a 7 than a 6 and she was able to identify that the medication had helped him be able to sit and focus for a little longer than previously, that even though he was still combative she has learned that by giving him some time to calm down he would sometimes eventually do whatever was requested, school had reported that he was actually paying attention a little more and was completing more of his work. I then asked given that she was a 7 on the scale, where would be good enough for her. She took some time to think about this and replied that she knows she will never be a 10 in terms of being satisfied with his behaviour, and said that she knows no kid can ever be perfect. She settled on one point higher on the scale as her "good enough." We were able to talk about what might move her a little higher on the scale over the next week or so, and she decided she needed to wait another week or so to see how the medication may help some more. She also decided to talk to the teacher about what was working in the classroom to help him complete his work to see if there was anything else she could be doing at home.

Conclusion

The SF way of communicating has given me an approach to my practice which enables me to meet clients and families exactly where they are, no matter how escalated, frustrated, and hopeless they appear. I no longer feel that crushing sense of responsibility that I have to make everything ok for them. I approach every interaction with the fundamental belief that at their core each individual is whole and with the strengths and resources needed to address the issues they face in their lives. My job is facilitating them remembering their wholeness, strengths, and resources, even if they seem unaware of them. I know this fundamental switch in my approach to my practice has enabled me to recover from my seemingly hopeless feelings of burnout in my work and approach each conversation I have with my families with curiosity, and feelings of confidence and competence. Do I still want to retire? Of course, I am nearing the age when I am ready for the next phase and adventure in my life. The difference is that I will not be leaving my career with a sense of failure and I know that I have shown up at work each day, and in each interaction with the clients and families, as my best self.

References

Akgul-Gundogdu, N. & Selcuk-Tosun, A. (2021). Examining the relationship between solution-focused thinking skills and self-efficacy levels of nursing students in Turkey. *Journal of Professional Nursing, 37*(4), 1180–1186.

Cook, E. (2022). The funnel of optimal functioning: A model coach education. *The Coaching Psychologist, 18*(2), 43–58.

Ge, M.W., Hu, F.H., Jia, Y.J., Tang, W., Zhang, W.Q., & Chen, H.L. (2023). Global prevalence of nursing burnout syndrome and temporal trends for the last 10 years: A meta-analysis of 94 studies covering over 30 countries. *Journal of Clinical Nursing, 32*(17–18), 5836–5854.

Johnson, B., Abraham, M., Conway, J., Simmons, L., Edgman-Levitan, S., Sodomka, P. et al. (2008). Partnering with patients and families to design a patient- and family-centered health care system: Recommendations and promising practices. Institute for Patient- and Family-Centered Care. Available at: https://www.ipfcc.org/resources/Roadmap.pdf

Kim, J.S., Brook, J., Liming, K.W., Park, I.Y., Akin, B.A., & Franklin, C. (2022). Randomized controlled trial study examining positive emotions and hope in solution-focused brief therapy with substance using parents involved in child welfare system. *International Journal of Systemic Therapy, 33*(1), 129–149.

Kim, J.S. & Franklin, C. (2015). Understanding emotional change in solution-focused brief therapy: Facilitating positive emotions. *Best Practices in Mental Health, 11*(1), 25–41.

King, G., Baldwin, P., Servais, M., & Moodie, S. (2022). Solution-focused coaching to support clinicians' professional development: An analysis of relational strategies and co-constructed outcomes. *Developmental Neurorehabilitation, 25*(3), 205–216.

King, G., Schwellnus, H., Servais, M., & Baldwin, P. (2019). Solution-focused coaching in pediatric rehabilitation: Investigating transformative experiences and outcomes for families. *Physical & Occupational Therapy in Pediatrics, 39*(1), 16–32.

Leiter, M.P. & Maslach, C. (2009). Nurse turnover: The mediating role of burnout. *Journal of Nursing Management, 17*(3), 331–339.

Luo, H., Cao, L., Yue, L., Peng, Z., Lei, X., Li, Z. et al. (2019). Solution-focused brief coaching: An exploratory study in nurses with burnout. *Journal of Systemic Therapies, 38*(4), 80–99.

Macdonald, A. (2007). *Solution-Focused Therapy: Theory, Research & Practice.* Sage Publications.

McPherson, A.C., Biddiss, E., Chen, L., Church, P.T., de Groot, J.F., Keenan, S. et al. (2019). Children and teens in charge of their health (CATCH): A protocol for a feasibility randomised controlled trial of solution-focused coaching to foster healthy lifestyles in childhood disability. *BMJ Open, 9*(3), article e025119.

Medina, A. & Beyebach, M. (2014). The impact of solution-focused training on profession-als' beliefs, practices and burnout of child protection workers in Tenerife Island. *Child Care in Practice, 20*(1), 7–36.

Remen, R.N. (1998). Whole patient whole doctor. *Advances in Mind-Body Medicine, 14*(1), 19–21.

Remen, R.N. (2008). Practicing a medicine of the whole person: An opportunity for healing. *Hematology/Ontology Clinics of North America, 22*(4), 767–773.

Theofanidis, D., Boukas, A., & Fountouki, A. (2022). A "new pandemic" at hand: Burnout of nursing staff. *International Journal of Caring Sciences, 15*(3), 2028–2035.

9 Solution-Focused Healthcare

Application and Benefits in Occupational Therapy

Amanda Musto

When I first encountered Solution-Focused Coaching, it was an Ah-Ha moment. As a community-based consultant for almost 10 years at the time, I had the privilege of working in a variety of settings: from fast-paced school consultations with teachers, to more personal consultations with new parents in their own homes. During this time, I experienced frustrated, burnt-out teachers sigh in exasperation, and repeatedly reject every recommendation I made, convinced nothing would work. I also witnessed amazing parents who did everything in their capacity to support their child's development, cry for hours after a follow-up visit with a doctor who emphasized their child's deficits and wanted them to do more. Personally, I experienced the disappointment and frustration of following up with a family or teacher, only to find that nothing, on the long list of recommendations I had worked hard to put together, had been tried. I was seen as the expert and expected to decide the right way forward and "fix the problem." For most of my career, that is what I tried to do. However, through all my experiences, frustrations, and successes, I felt there was more to my role than coming in and telling people what was wrong, and how to fix it. There was value simply in acknowledging, and validating the lived experience of individuals, as well as their strength and resilience as they managed their circumstances.

When I discovered humanistic and solution-focused coaching, the means to practise in a manner consistent with my own values became apparent. I realized that coming in and asserting my expertise was not and is not helpful, as this minimizes the expertise of the client, and fails to acknowledge the efforts and successes that have already occurred. Instead, my real work is to elicit, amplify, and reinforce the strengths and resources of my clients, in order to develop their agency as the authorities of their own healthcare journeys. I felt I finally had permission, backed by research and evidence-based models, to support how I intuitively wanted to practise and engage with my clients.

In my current role as a consultant to daycare environments, I often enter into situations where power dynamics are well established and where multiple ideas and personalities are in conflict. I see my role as a Solution-Focused Health Care Coach (SFHCC) and an Occupational Therapist (OT) as helping to shift my clients' attention away from deficits and unwanted "behaviours," to their strengths, the child's strengths, and towards a more meaningful way forward that is unique to them. Both SFHCC and OT roles bring with them a strengths-based lens that

DOI: 10.4324/9781003414490-11

can help support my clients to make this shift. As an SFHCC, I can use questions to elicit, amplify, and reinforce clients' strengths and resources so they are able to recognize, acknowledge, and trust their own observations and strategies that have worked in the past. With my OT training, I can validate many of their observations and successes through theories and models. The combination of both approaches allows me to help the client realize they are already intuitively supporting the child in many ways. Such an approach provides a foundation from which we can build and move forward collaboratively. As a result, I am able to work with the team and include their expertise and observations to create new strategies that meet their needs in a more meaningful way.

Overall, providing humanistic healthcare enables the client to recognize their own resources. Every healthcare encounter is an opportunity for the coach-clinician to model and reinforce that the client is the expert in their own life and healthcare journey. This coaching approach enables the clinician to become an ally and collaborator, supporting and nurturing clients' agency. In this way, the humanistic approach allowed me to move from being a fixer to a facilitator and collaborator (see Figure 9.1). By amplifying and reinforcing the client's strengths and resources, their resilience and confidence to work through not only what they are focusing on in that moment, but whatever may come in the future, increases.

When completing my SFHCC training, I was amazed how the principles of Humanistic and Solution-Focused Coaching could be utilized in so many different contexts, which is evident by the publication of this book. It was also fascinating to see how each individual used the questions and principles of solution-focused coaching (SFC) in their own way to fit their strengths and roles. Below, I hope to highlight some practical strategies I have been able to implement in my practice and the difference this has made.

HEALING VS FIXING

Fixing	Healing
• Client is a problem to fix	• Client is whole
• Clinician is expert	• Client is the expert of their own lived experience
• Client is dependent	• Client is autonomous
• Directive and authoritative	• Relational
• Emphasis is on what is broken	• Remembering wholeness

Figure 9.1 Healing vs Fixing

Pre-Session Change Questions

One of the first and most significant changes that I made in my practice was contracting with my clients through pre-session change questions. This begins even before my consultation starts. When responding to a referral I ask: "What will be most helpful for us to focus on during our consultation?" I often couple this with a constraint: "given that this is a one-time consultation," or "given that we have 45 minutes together," or "given this is a group care environment, what would be most helpful for us to discuss, focus on, or explore together?" As a pre-session change question, I am not expecting a response until we meet in person. I encourage the referral source to go back to their team, and the family to decide this together. Often, a referral is made because everyone agrees there is a "problem," but less often do teams know specifically what they would like instead. Through pre-session change questions, I am gently shifting their focus from the problem to a desired outcome, and helping stakeholders to come to a consensus before the consultation. *Of note, I am making a positive assumption that the group has the strength and resources to work together and come to a consensus.* By asking these types of pre-session change questions, I am respecting the stakeholders' authority and expertise in their lived experience, and empowering them to identify what they need in the moment. Therefore, not only am I establishing a focus for the consultation, I'm laying the foundation for a collaborative experience, by reinforcing that I believe they know what is most important to focus on to make meaningful change in their specific context.

Listening for Understanding

One of the most humbling lessons in my SFHCC training was the concept of listening to understand. I had always considered myself to be a good listener; however, I realized I was constantly filtering what I heard through my clinical bias. I was deciding what was important and where to focus. I decided what the problem was, where to start, and how the problem was going to be solved. When what you've deemed is important is incongruent with what the client wants to focus on, a tension and dynamic can be created. As opposed to collaboration, the discussion can become defensive and oppositional.

Listening to understand and following the client's lead requires flexibility and the ability to relinquish control, which can be challenging. However, this is how we can truly create a spirit of collaboration. The humanistic approach has helped me to be truly curious, without an agenda, to listen to what might be behind what the client is saying, as deeper meanings are not always stated. Preserving the language your client uses during the discussion is especially powerful, as it demonstrates you are deeply listening to what they are saying and not simply filtering and interpreting their words to form your own conclusions. Listening to understand, without judgement or bias, demonstrates compassion, and allows you to meet your client where they are in the moment. When you are able to be in the moment with your client, you are better able to lead from behind; following their lead by asking questions to elicit, amplify, and reinforce the strengths and observations they've demonstrated and shared.

Noticing and Reinforcing

There is a vulnerability to seeking help, which can lead to a client's defences being high, and a heightened stress response. Simply noticing and acknowledging what clients are doing well, and recognizing the difference their efforts made for the child, reinforces their skills and expertise. Genuine acknowledgement, without exaggeration or platitudes, is an indirect compliment, and can help the client feel seen and heard. Reinforcing and nurturing your client's strengths reduces this vulnerability or insecurity they may have been feeling. This allows for a more collaborative conversation. Noticing and reinforcing can be completed through observation or by listening for their strengths and insights when they speak and reflecting this back to them, for example: "I noticed how you got down to their level when you spoke to them, and how they smiled and looked at you when you did that. It was such a nice moment of connection. How did you come up with that strategy?" Through modelling and highlighting what is already working, clients are inclined to follow that lead and identify strategies that have been working for them, even just a little. Problem talk will naturally arise, it is in our nature; however, by continuing to notice and reinforce the client's strengths, a positive feedback loop can be created to steer the conversation in a solution-focused direction.

Asking for Permission

Before offering any clinical expertise or education, I check in and ask for permission. For example, I might ask, "Would it be helpful if I provided some education around stages of readiness for eating?" This is a simple yet powerful way to reinforce that your clients are the experts in their healthcare journey and know what will be most helpful to them. It follows the collaborative nature of the consultation, and allows you to lead your client from behind.

Navigating the Tension between Clinical Expertise and a Stance of Curiosity – Holding Space for Two Realities

When providing education, I will infuse my explanation with clinical examples I observed, or the client shared. This is an opportunity to reflect back their observations and experiences and reframe them in an objective and respectful way. By using their lived-experience, it makes the education more tangible and meaningful. The goal is not to imply that their perspective is wrong, or convince them that you are right, just simply to reflect back what you were told and provide a different way to interpret their observations. When done without judgement or a clear bias and agenda, clients are more open to a shift in perspective. For example, I might explain that the child is chewing on objects to help self-regulate, instead of seeking attention, or purposefully causing destruction. I'll use examples of what I observed and anecdotes that they shared to help illustrate a different picture, for instance. "I observed when the classroom became loud, they started biting on their sleeves. Have you noticed any other patterns or times they will bite more frequently?" There are often many ah-ha moments during this reframing part of the discussion. Clients often recount other instances when the behaviour occurred, and are able to make the reframe themselves. Or even better, they are able to recount when a strategy worked, and why, based on this new education and perspective. This is an opportunity to reinforce and affirm this new understanding and perspective. Importantly, if they are not able to see this new perspective, or do not agree, that is okay. By reflecting their observations and experiences back to them, you are still listening to understand and noticing and reinforcing as outlined above. By sharing your expertise without trying to convince or pressure them, you are continuing to respect their expertise as someone who knows their environment, child, and lived experience best. Such an approach allows you to maintain a collaborative and respectful foundation for future engagement. It also plants a seed for different perspectives respectfully, and without pressure, that they can revisit if and when they choose.

Collaborative Recommendations

When exploring recommendations to move forward, I start by highlighting what is already working and encourage them to simply continue doing more of that. This reduces mental stress and burden on the client, as it highlights that they are already moving in the right direction, and simply continuing to do what they are doing is enough. Once this positive reinforcement is provided, I ask if they have any ideas about how they might be able to integrate these existing strategies into different parts of their day or routine. Allowing the client to take the lead is essential, as they are the experts in their environment and lived experience, and they know best how to make these adaptations fit their environment. By taking such an approach, we are able to broaden their capacity and confidence, and build on these established strengths; therefore, recommendations are less intimidating as we are building on established strengths and strategies, and not starting from scratch.

Goal Setting

Often, the concerns expressed are around reducing unwanted "behaviours." In SFC, the absence of something is not a goal. As a result, the client must identify *what they would like instead* (of the problem) and then work towards that as a goal. When providing my clinical expertise, I often reframe the "behaviour" as a communication or as a strategy for self-regulation. Understanding that the child is trying to communicate or meet an unmet need helps guide adults to understand what the child is seeking and therefore helps give a direction to what they would like. I often give examples of general strategies that can redirect a child; however, I always acknowledge that it is their space, and therefore the chosen activity or strategy needs to work for them. By offering general strategies and leaving space for disagreement, discussion, or infusion of their own interpretation, strategies unique to the child emerge – strategies that I could never have generated on my own.

Additionally, if strategies and ideas are internally generated, they are more likely to be meaningful and therefore achievable.

Session Close

When ending a session, I like to ask some variation of, "what strategy are you most excited to try first," "which strategy did you feel will be most beneficial," "what was the most helpful part of our discussion today," or "which strategy do you think the child will be most excited for." This is a great way to end the session as it allows them to already start envisioning the changes in the classroom as well as the difference these changes will make for them and the child. It is always interesting and humbling to hear the responses, as often their responses are not what I anticipate – highlighting, again, only they can truly know what is most helpful and meaningful for them.

The Funnel of Optimal Functioning

Although this is not explicitly a strategy, it is a valuable representation of how the above strategies work so well throughout the session, and how to navigate the conversation. Generally, clients begin at the bottom of the funnel: as outlined above, they feel vulnerable and defensive. They are stuck in problem-focused thinking, and are not yet in the mind space to see the progress they are already making, never mind the next steps forward. Through listening for understanding, and validating their expertise and lived experience through asking for permission, holding space, highlighting what is working, indirect compliments, and leading from behind, the client moves up the funnel. This is seen in the energy and increased participation in the session. It's a tangible energy shift as the conversation progresses. If the energy remains low, you may need to spend more time moving them up the funnel before you start collaborating on recommendations or next steps.

For me, moving the client up the funnel is as important as, if not more important than, the recommendations themselves. When a client leaves a consultation at the top of the behaviour funnel, they are more motivated to follow through, and they feel more capable and empowered, able to access resources, and able to see solutions. A consultation without movement up the funnel would result in a client feeling burdened, overwhelmed, or guilty about another list of recommendations. Helping move a client up the behaviour funnel is the mechanism through which coaches are able to nurture their client's autonomy and ability to be more resourceful and resilient, now and in the future. This is the value of embedding solution-focused questions and humanistic dialogue in my practice.

Clinician Benefits

Embedding these ideas, principles, and strategies into my practice has not only benefited my clients, it has had a positive impact on me as well. The mutual benefits of SFC allow for an effective and sustainable way of practising, which can be insulating from fatigue and burn-out. Below, I hope to extol a few of the many positive changes I have experienced.

Previously, when I decided the focus and what needed to be done in a consultation, the conversation would often get pulled in multiple directions. I felt much of our time and my energy was spent trying to keep us on topic. I would feel frustrated that the client was not listening to me and trusting me to know what needed to be done. By the end of the consultation, there were multiple topics discussed and only superficial strategies to show for our time. Conversely, when the client is able to identify the focus of the consultation, we are able to efficiently and thoroughly explore a topic that is most meaningful and helpful to them. As a result, clinically, I feel I am better able to support my clients by co-creating recommendations that are individualized to them and will make a material impact in their lives. Providing quality care to clients and enabling them to make positive changes in their lives is an extremely gratifying experience.

Humanistic care replaces the traditional power dynamic of the clinician as the expert and the client as the learner. Instead, the client and clinician come together as equals, each with our own strengths and knowledge, to work collaboratively towards a common goal. It's a very subtle yet powerful shift to move from seeing yourself as the "fixer," who holds all the answers, to a collaborator, who provides education, facilitates the conversation, and nurtures the client's existing strengths and resources. This shift relieved the immense pressure I felt as a clinician. You are no longer burdened with the responsibility of your client's "problems" and how to solve them, as the problems are no longer the focus. Your attention starts to shift to all the good that is happening, even just a little bit; that they managed to show up for the appointment, that they care enough to attend, that they have insight and resources to access your services. When you start to look for the positives, they continue to manifest, especially when you elicit these strengths from your client. Simple questions such as, "How did you manage to get to today's appointment despite the challenges involved in leaving the house?" With this lens, you can then support your client to see these strengths within themselves and instill in them the confidence that they can continue to make positive changes.

Practising in this way can be quite energizing as opposed to draining. Admittedly, it does take a lot of energy to be present in the moment, listen with genuine curiosity, and facilitate the conversations in a solution-focused format, yet the result is constantly rewarding.

Lastly, it is difficult to describe, but when practising in a solution-focused manner, I feel a tangible change in the energy in the room. As discussed previously, clients can feel vulnerable when seeking help, which can cause defensiveness. Providing prescriptive advice can exacerbate this vulnerability and lead to tension or rejection of ideas. This was an energy I knew too well, and I often felt defeated when my client rejected my ideas or didn't follow through. The key is genuine curiosity and willingness to follow the client's lead and not just listening to respond. Humanistic care acknowledges the client's expertise and encourages collaboration at its core. When people notice their opinions and thoughts are not only welcomed, but also valued, the energy of the conversation shifts. A positive momentum can be created by building on each other's insights and ideas. It is a welcome and contagious energy. At times, the room can become giddy, wanting to share an idea, or a new connection they made about what was discussed. There can also be tears, because they feel seen and acknowledged for the hard work they are already doing. Overall, it feels like a pleasant conversation among peers who are interested and invested in the same outcomes. Clients leave feeling empowered and motivated to make the changes that are important and meaningful for them, as opposed to feeling overwhelmed, burdened, or discouraged.

I am so grateful for the initial training I received that introduced me to SFC and for the opportunities I've had to continue to learn and develop my practice as a Certified Solution-Focused Coach and Facilitator. Being able to practise in a way that aligns with my values as a human and as a clinician is so fulfilling. Being able to practise among colleagues, and within an organization that supports the same values of humanistic care, is even more enabling and enriching. I'm humbled and inspired to be able to share my knowledge and experience with my students and colleagues who are curious and want to learn more. I feel a renewed sense of purpose in my work, to enable my clients not only through education, but through acknowledging their strength and resilience and reflecting this back to them. There is a great satisfaction in seeing my clients acknowledge and embrace their abilities and authority to move forward in a way that is meaningful to them.

Engaging in a humanistic fashion is not limited to healthcare, but can be applied to all relationships and interactions. When we can be curious, and listen to understand, we connect and demonstrate compassion to our clients, colleagues, family members, and even strangers. Connecting through compassion and respect for one another's knowledge and lived experience has deepened my practice and my relationships in general. There is meaning and beauty in this connection and I'm grateful I now understand this value and make it a priority in my practice and life.

Section Three

Lived Experience

10 A Discussion of Solution-Focused Praxis through a Lived Experience of Disability

Wesley Magee-Saxton

At this point in the journey, over the course of many chapters, a clear picture has been painted on what solution-focused work is and what its implications are. In this chapter, I will delve into the past to explore how the need for this program developed and why it is important for us to keep one foot in acknowledgement and one foot in possibility, as we strive for change in healthcare. I am a white 23-year-old disabled and non-binary person currently in training to receive my solution-focused coaching certification. In this chapter, I hope to share the salient parts of my journey through the Canadian healthcare system as a queer wheelchair user with cerebral palsy and a burgeoning humanistic, solution-focused reframe.

My reality as a disabled individual means that I have been intertwined with the healthcare system from birth and my survival has been a struggle in advocacy. In that same breath, the privilege that I hold as a white person is incredibly important to acknowledge as I speak throughout this chapter and to illustrate that privilege does make navigation easier (Columbia Law School, 2017).

From the moment I was born, my family's world was turned on its head. We were thrust into closer proximity with the healthcare system than most can imagine and I was already being pathologized in my first breaths of life. In time, we would learn that the healthcare system is oriented as a pyramid structure and that the majority of interactions with that system conditioned us to be passive receivers of information doled out by those at the top of the pyramid, those with power and authority. Let me be very clear, I do not mean to disregard expertise; I only mean to illustrate that there was little to no space given for me or my family to offer our own lived experience as experts of our own lives. I was constantly seen as a problem to be fixed and instances where I was seen as a whole person were few and far between, especially when I was younger. As I have grown older, this has become somewhat easier, yet I constantly feel dissonance between seeking a humanistic healing approach and being given one that seeks to fix me instead.

How did we get to the system I have outlined above? What are the roots of this pathology-based praxis with only a few making efforts to resist it? An answer lies in viewing our history with a critical disability lens. The origins of our modern healthcare system can be seen in the thinking processes associated with The Age of Enlightenment (Berg, 2020). It was a time of great categorization and classification

DOI: 10.4324/9781003414490-13

which resulted in marginalized people and any deviation from the norm being seen as a problem to be fixed or eradicated (Berg, 2020). This type of thinking resulted in a modern healthcare system that resembled a machine. This machine was designed to take in "broken" people and spit them out as fixed problems. In such a mechanized system, there is no room for the acknowledgement of patients as whole beings because there is an overreliance on a transactional approach.

This dogmatic doctrine is inherently problem-focused and only reinforces the negative neural pathways that much of human nature tends to be drawn towards (Vaish et al., 2008). This creates a never-ending cycle of a downward spiral that causes individuals and communities to lose trust in their own experience. Seeing humans as equations to be solved and classified gives the system only a false image of success. There are countless people who fall through the cracks, all because our current system is ingrained in this authoritarian power structure as a holdover from previous centuries.

The main objective of solution-focused work is to take the authoritarian structure of our current system and reshape it, levelling the playing field between professional and client. The goal is to create a structure that is circular, like the ripples in a pond. Such a shape captures the constant movement inherent in human interactions and allows healthcare relationships to become collaborative and relational, existing in the shared space between professional and client that is upheld equally by both parties. Instead of seeing patients as problems to be fixed, solution-focused work places emphasis on inherent wholeness. This is a shift that is incredibly simple in concept and yet requires practised discipline to implement as we have to do the difficult work of extricating ourselves from the above-mentioned system.

The easiest example to exemplify the necessity of ripple effect in my own experience comes from navigating the power dynamics of attendant care. I require a great deal of attendant care for daily living tasks. These tasks can include everything from dressing, showering, and going to the washroom, to meal prep and basic house-cleaning. Access to attendant care dictates whether I can live by myself, engage with my community, and even go to work. Without attendant care, I would need constant assistance from friends and family to access the world from an electric wheelchair, in a body that deals with fine motor issues and chronic pain. My reality makes this type of care a non-negotiable prerequisite for having any quality of life. Having proper humanistic care of this nature enables me to have full control over my existence.

As outlined above, it is very easy to see how imperative attendant care support is required in my life. This also means that negative experiences from attendant care sometimes seem impossible to escape, especially when attendants are present in my home from the moment I open my eyes, until they close again at the end of the day. Those who utilize attendant care as a tributary of our healthcare system are not afforded the luxury of being able to wake up prior to interacting with staff. I have had many challenging experiences with personal support workers who did not see me as human. Attendants saw me as a task to complete, a booking to finish, or in the worst cases, a science project to be studied. They took on the role of authority in my care and did not permit me to insert the wealth of experience that I have as the sole recipient of my own care into the equation. Instead, they dismissed any input I had to make the process of my care easier, safer, and more comfortable for them. They stuck dogmatically to a one-size-fits-all practice, which in the end resulted in mental and physical stress, as well as pain. This created a constant downward spiral for not only myself, but also the staff involved. No one was happy and no one was looking forward to the bookings.

However, there is a solution-focused theme that threads itself through this chapter and the work I now do: one foot in acknowledgement and one foot in possibility. Using the lens of attendant care, this concept is enacted when both parties recognize the importance of the training that attendant care staff receive to keep both the client and the staff safe, as well as staff collaborating with the client to figure out what works best for them – even if it requires a deviation from basic training. Personal support staff who operate through a humanistic lens employ tenets of solution-focused work without even realizing it. The atmosphere is generative, welcoming, and safe. Processes are built through a lens that broadens and builds out to create the perfect bookings. There is social contracting throughout and constraints are seen as a positive guide rather than a challenge. Power is shared through a symbiotic game of give and take within self-direction. I have found that humour and fun even make their way into these humanistic bookings without sacrificing the necessary levels of professionalism.

The difference is evident when attendant care is infused with solution-focused practice. The effect on my life is immeasurable and truly moves me towards both self-actualization and community actualization. A solution-focused frame makes the difference between dreading attendant care bookings and gentle peace for all involved. It reduces the workload for both myself and the staff. One can see the seamless integration of acknowledgement in conjunction with possibility when the professional experience of the attendant is honoured, and it does not supersede the expertise of the client. The same applies to solution-focused work in general within healthcare. When the client is trusted to be the author of their own story, it takes the onus off the clinician to be the eternal and all-knowing expert. This practice reduces burnout and improves interpersonal outcomes.

Solution-focused frames must be looked at as an absolute necessity, especially when working with those with disabilities and other identities marginalized by the healthcare system. Quite often, training forgets how varied and diverse our realities are and views us only as monoliths. As illustrated at the beginning of this chapter, as disabled people we know this and recognize the harm our healthcare system has caused for hundreds of years. In addition, it is impossible for training to cover every single variable identity that clinicians may encounter. Relying on the expertise of the client regarding their own lives and experience is the only way clinicians can accurately know the reality of the client. Any assumption otherwise is not only arrogant, but it is also simply incorrect.

In my past, I once worked with a care staff individual who was part of my daily shower booking. It goes without saying that warm showers are nearly universally loved in some way by everyone. They are definitely one of my favourite parts of the day. This care staff told me that they were getting wet in the shower when help-ing me and as such would only be giving me military style showers. This meant that I was soaped up without running water and briefly hosed down (often with cold water) once that had been completed. It was miserable and I tried to communicate as such. Every attempt at resolution was shut down by the staff, citing that they were the expert and they had other bookings to get to so I just had to deal with it. This went on for a long time and I began to dread bookings with this individual, feeling that I was making no progress and being robbed of something that was important to me. One morning, I took them aside and asked what they enjoyed about warm showers. It was like something clicked in their brain and I was seen as a human who wanted a moment of enjoyment and warmth, rather than a task to be done. From that point on, I was able to collaborate with them on finding a solu-tion that worked for us and accomplished what we both wanted. All it took was the realization of commonality between the two of us.

Perhaps the most unexpected example of a similar circumstance was a staff sud-denly refusing to help me put on my service dog's identifier jacket after years of doing so. They claimed that I had been forcing them to do it for years when they didn't want to and were afraid of dogs in general, despite the fact that they never communicated with me as such. My poor dog was so confused as she is always happy to see the staff and would never hurt a fly. After speaking with the staff, I learned that they were afraid of dogs because they'd been hurt by one in the past. Now it was my turn to honour the staff as the expert of their own experience. I had to work with the constraints of that fear despite the fact that I still needed assistance putting on my dog's uniform. In the end, I worked with community supports to find alternate ways to put on my service dog's uniforms when that particular staff was helping me in the morning. After that relatively small collaborative adjustment, the quality of our bookings together increased tenfold because everyone felt safe and supported. The power dynamic was equalized and replaced by the ripple effect mentioned above. Both of our days became easier.

I paired these examples together to highlight how different actions were re-quired to find resolutions to these issues. The staff had to trust me to be the expert of my own experience and I also had to trust and honour the expertise of theirs to be truly relational. As stated earlier in this chapter, there is room to honour the expertise of every party without one superseding the other. This work is designed to be malleable enough to fit into any shape that a shared space might occupy. One of the most important lessons I learned from both of these experiences was to ask with curiosity. This step can often open many unforeseen pathways even when one occupied a position of compliance at the bottom of the historical power structure.

It is worth noting that all of the outcomes I mentioned above are unquestionably revolutionary and yet only require small shifts; extremely subtle change in attitudes of the minutiae of day-to-day attendant care. These changes are very achievable in their execution and their effect ripples through almost every aspect of my life. By its very nature, solution-focused work begs practitioners to engage on the level of the micro to affect the macro. This work is highly successful in achieving very large goals because it does not shy away from the reality of them. It knows that in order to achieve those lofty goals, we must do so in stages and it trusts clients as the experts to define what stages work for them. No matter the size of our goal, solution-focused work trusts that we have the resources to achieve it. This trust is why we can utilize the work to create a roadmap to something as small as wanting to figure out how to meal prep more to something as large as restructuring an antiquated healthcare system on the systemic level.

In this chapter, I have used my primary experience with attendant care as the main example scenario of the application of solution-focused work. It is also worth noting that these notions can be applied to every aspect of the healthcare system, whether in paediatric or adult services across the entire spectrum. There must always be room for client expertise in every scenario. It is our job as healthcare professionals to walk the line of acknowledgement and possibility.

Through showcasing the microcosm of the singular thread of my experience in this system that has been so utterly pervasive in my life, I hope to have shown readers of this text that there is a pathway forward. There is a way to find cracks in systems that we must participate in and for us to be the organisms that rebuild them. Many of the fundamental changes spoken about in this chapter require such small changes to yield incredible results. When our healthcare system dedicates itself to change on both a micro and macro level, we will be able to develop a healthcare system that is fundamentally as alive as we are as individuals. Outdated teachings from the past will be shed and, rather than acting as a machine, our healthcare system will be able to symbiotically respond to those who need access to it. We will be able to build an ecosystem that is able to better handle the stresses and demands of modern healthcare without sacrificing the need to cradle the story of every client. When clients move from the position of passive receivers to authors of their own stories, they become just as important as any clinical member of the healthcare team. Solution-focused work will help clinicians and clients to weave a new system together that disregards old hierarchies and leaves all involved with a lasting sense of wholeness and energy.

This shift to humanistic-focused healthcare will take time and effort. It will meet resistance as the old systems are so ingrained in our neural pathways that it will be difficult for everyone to shift away. As stated in multiplicity throughout the chapter, small actions can be massive in their results. Many professionals have witnessed what I have outlined above and balked at the prospect of making the shift. Just as this work uses the Broaden and Build theory (Fredrickson, 2004) on an individual level within sessions, the very nature of the work itself is ingrained in growth. I speak from experience, as I have seen the work itself be my biggest supporter and believe fully that that same theory can also be applied on a macro level. A garden cannot be sewn and reaped within the same breath. We have to start by planting the seeds in our communities. When we place our trust in humanistic, solution-focused work, we can replace a tired machine with an ever-evolving organism that sees all of us as whole.

References

Berg, S. (2020). *A Cultural History of Disability*, Vol. 4: *In the Long Eighteenth Century* (C. Gabbard & S.B. Mintz, eds). Bloomsbury Academic.
Columbia Law School. (2017, June 8). Kimberlé crenshaw on intersectionality, more than two decades later. Available at: https://www.law.columbia.edu/news/archive/kimberle-crenshaw-intersectionality-more-two-decades-later
Fredrickson, B.L. (2004). The broaden-and-build theory of positive emotions. *Philosophical Transactions of the Royal Society of London. Series B: Biological Sciences*, *359*(1449), 1367–1377.
Vaish, A., Grossmann, T., & Woodward, A. (2008). Not all emotions are created equal: The negativity bias in social-emotional development. *Psychological Bulletin*, *134*(3), 383–403.

11 Embracing a Humanistic Solution-Focused Approach

Implications for Living with Cerebral Palsy for Me and My Family

Nikky Henderson

The humanistic, solution-focused approach has been a transformative force in shaping my identity. It's been a journey of self-discovery, realizing my wholeness, and recognizing the intricacies of my existence across various facets of life. In this space, I share my experiences with this approach that has fundamentally altered my perspective.

My Story

I am Nikky Henderson, entering the world on a crisp fall day in a Toronto hospital during the 1990s. My odyssey commenced at 29 weeks, a significant 11 weeks before my anticipated due date. My mother faced daunting challenges during her pregnancy, enduring complete bed rest. The isolation of nine months, with hopes pinned on reaching 28 weeks for foetal viability, became her reality. My premature arrival, 11 weeks early, wasn't entirely unexpected. Potential complications, including challenges in communication and mobility, were listed by the doctor. Adoption was even suggested due to perceived complexities. The *Humanistic approach* emphasizes the fundamental principle that everyone is *whole*. Starting life already perceived as less than whole can have devastating impacts. Similarly, in solution-focused work, we straddle acknowledgement and possibility. While the medical model predicts quality of life based on statistics, it fails to recognize the limitless potential within individuals.

In my early years, I met most developmental milestones, barring some physical limitations. Despite being an adorable, babbling baby, walking posed a challenge. Doctor consultations yielded resistance, advising my mother to wait. A pivotal turning point emerged only after seeking a second opinion, leading to a diagnosis that became crucial for early intervention and eventual thriving.

Reflecting on my journey, the weight of labels in our systems becomes apparent. A diagnosis or label can open doors to crucial resources, but also has the potential to confine individuals within predefined boxes. Labels aim for efficiency, assuming that if you fit a particular box, you share similarities with others. Yet, even among those with similar traits, diversity prevails. At the age of 5, I was diagnosed with Cerebral Palsy (CP), a two-letter word that would accompany me throughout life, bringing both wonderful and painful memories. While CP is a well-researched

DOI: 10.4324/9781003414490-14

condition, the label can lead to assumptions. The impact of labels is evident in how society perceives and interacts with individuals with disabilities. Despite having a mild, sometimes invisible disability, assumptions about intelligence or competency persist. Statements like, "You talk so well," or "You would never know over the phone or email that you have a disability," reveal a mistaken correlation between disability and cognitive ability. It's crucial to recognize that while some individuals with disabilities may face cognitive challenges, generalizing this to all is unfair.

Reflecting on my journey as a young person navigating the world with a physical disability, I can't ignore the prevalence of deficit-based language in healthcare and educational spaces. The repetition of "she can't do that" or "that would be too difficult" has left a profound impact. As the humanistic model highlights, words have the power to shape our brains, and hearing the word "can't" can significantly influence one's self-image.

Society often imposes boxes, defining expectations for individuals. Whether it's gender expectations, racial stereotypes, or assumptions about disabilities, these limiting statements persist. I proudly identify as a Black woman with a disability, challenging these constraints passed down both explicitly and implicitly.

My Family's Story with Me

The humanistic, solution-focused approach has profoundly influenced my family's dynamics, offering a framework and language that supports a deeper understanding of my *agency* and *wholeness*. One pivotal shift has been in our overall perception of wholeness, moving away from viewing me solely through the lens of my diagnoses. Instead, I am recognized as a composite of various elements that contribute to my unique story.

During healthcare appointments, these constituent elements are now integral to our conversations, allowing me to be acknowledged beyond my diagnoses. This shift towards recognizing the entirety of who I am originated in our home, initiated through initial discussions exploring the elements that define me. Although I lacked the language to comprehend it at the time, the humanistic principles were gradually weaving themselves into the fabric of my narrative.

Navigating the healthcare system often involves advocating for resources, necessitating the retelling of one's story, and, at times, overemphasizing challenges to secure appropriate support. A simple acknowledgement of my *strengths and resources* within this process would have significantly boosted my overall self-confidence.

In reflecting on our unique journeys, particularly in comparison to my younger sibling, who is 11 years my junior and does not have a disability, it becomes evident how *transformative* this approach has been. Embracing the humanistic principles has opened our eyes to the importance of recognizing and valuing everyone's journey, fostering a more inclusive and supportive family dynamic.

Family serves as the foundation, offering support and understanding during the highs and lows. In my family, comprised of myself, my mum, my younger brother, my dad, and stepdad, we function as a cohesive team, especially when it comes to navigating the complex terrain of healthcare. Our family dynamic is a unique blend of personalities, each member contributing to the collective journey. With an age gap of 11 years between my brother and me, our sibling relationship is a classic dance of the older sister and younger brother, complete with the usual banter. Being the older sibling, I often find myself in the role of the bossy elder, but within this seemingly typical relationship, there are subtleties that define our bond.

One aspect that stands out is the collaborative effort we put into overcoming daily challenges. Tasks that may seem ordinary to others become significant for me due to issues with balance. It's not just about being the bossy older sister; it's about recognizing and appreciating the unique dynamics that exist within our relationship. Whether it's carrying items that are difficult for me to handle or assisting me in navigating stairs, each family member plays a role in enhancing my quality of life.

Amid the challenges of healthcare, my mother has been the primary family member attending appointments, providing unwavering support and additional information when needed. However, this has unintentionally led to misconceptions and questioning from healthcare professionals. Doctors often wonder why my mother is the sole attendee, prompting assumptions about her marital status and my family structure.

The reality, hidden behind these assumptions, lies in the nature of specialist appointments. These crucial healthcare sessions are often scheduled months in advance, making it challenging for other family members to synchronize time off work or school. It's imperative to shed light on the assumptions made when only one parent attends an appointment, especially considering the racial stereotypes that further complicate the perception. As a Black woman, I've encountered inquiries about the presence of my father at home, perpetuating harmful stereotypes based on appearances.

When you have a disability, receiving care often means that attention is directed towards your accompanying support individual rather than yourself. In the context of my CP diagnosis, people tend to focus solely on the deficits, making assumptions about my abilities and communication skills. The prevailing stereotype suggests that I must be in a wheelchair and incapable of clearly expressing my expectations or ideas.

This tendency to direct questions and concerns towards accompanying support individuals not only undermines my autonomy, but also leads to a demoralizing experience. Instead of being an active participant in my healthcare journey, I often feel like a bystander, disconnected from my own narrative. In the realm of humanistic healthcare, the importance of patients taking an active role in discussions and understanding their own journey is emphasized. Making assumptions about individuals, places, and things denies them autonomy, a crucial aspect of *person-centred care*.

Adopting a humanistic lens has been transformative in how I view my relationships, particularly with my sibling. Rather than focusing solely on perceived limitations, this perspective allows me to appreciate the richness of our connection. Beyond the occasional dependence on my younger sibling, I acknowledge the myriad ways in which I contribute to his growth and development.

This shift in perspective emphasizes the holistic nature of our relationships, moving beyond challenges to recognize the opportunities for mutual support and growth. It's a journey of self-discovery and understanding, not just for me, but also for each family member involved. As we navigate the complexities of life, health, and relationships, the humanistic approach serves as a guiding principle, reminding us of the importance of empathy, understanding, and active participation in our own narratives.

In the vast landscape of *family dynamics* and healthcare experiences, each nuance contributes to the unique tapestry of life. From the intricacies of sibling relationships to the challenges of healthcare stereotypes, this exploration aims to shed light on the multifaceted nature of our journey. As we navigate through life, embracing a humanistic approach allows us to redefine relationships, challenge assumptions, and actively participate in our own stories.

The Healthcare System and Person-Centred Care

In reflecting on my journey through the healthcare system, it's crucial to acknowledge the negative experiences that have shaped my perspective. However, it's equally important to carve out space to celebrate the success stories and individuals within the healthcare space who have made a positive impact on my life.

The healthcare system, despite its noble intentions, often falls short in providing a truly holistic experience for individuals with unique needs such as mine. Negative encounters, ranging from stereotyping to unintentional insensitivity, have left lasting impressions. These instances have fuelled my desire not only to share the challenges, but also to shed light on the brighter side of my healthcare journey.

One of the recurring issues I've faced is the tendency to reduce my identity to my condition. When the focus is solely on CP and related needs during appointments, it fosters a sense of being seen as a set of symptoms rather than as a complete person. This narrow perspective overlooks the rich tapestry of my individuality. Amid the challenges, there have been shining moments of success. These are instances where healthcare professionals took the time to see me beyond my diagnosis and delve into the person behind the medical history. These individuals stand out for their commitment to understanding me as a whole individual, recognizing that my interests and aspirations extend beyond the confines of my condition.

One striking example involves healthcare providers who went the extra mile to inquire about my interests, hobbies, and daily life outside the scope of CP. Instead of rushing through appointments solely focused on medical needs, they took the time to engage with me on a personal level. Questions like, "What does Nikky like to do in her spare time?" and "What does a typical day look like for you?" were asked, creating an environment where I felt seen and valued as an individual. These seemingly simple questions made a profound difference in my healthcare experience. By acknowledging and exploring facets of my life unrelated to my condition, healthcare professionals demonstrated a genuine interest in me as a person. It was more than just medical care; it was a recognition of my humanity.

This approach not only fostered a *positive doctor–patient relationship*, but also contributed to a more comprehensive understanding of my needs. It allowed for tailored and *personalized care* that considered not only the medical aspects of my condition, but also the broader context of my life. The success stories within my healthcare journey underscore the significance of nuanced interactions. These are the instances where the healthcare system transcended its clinical obligations to embrace the human aspect of care. By taking the time to understand me as an individual, healthcare professionals contributed to a more *positive and empowering* healthcare experience.

As I share these success stories, my intention is not to downplay the challenges, but to highlight the transformative power of *personalized, humanistic care*. It serves as a beacon, guiding the way towards a healthcare system that sees individuals not as a collection of symptoms, but as unique, multifaceted human beings. It is my hope that these success stories serve as a catalyst for change within the healthcare system. Advocating for a more comprehensive approach that values personal connections alongside medical expertise is crucial. Recognizing the individual behind the diagnosis is not just a nicety; it is fundamental to fostering a healthcare environment that is truly *person-centred*.

My healthcare journey has been marked by both challenges and successes. While negative experiences have highlighted the shortcomings in the system, the positive encounters with healthcare professionals who took the time to know me as an individual exemplify the transformative impact of humanistic care. By *amplifying* these success stories, I aim to contribute to a broader conversation about redefining healthcare to encompass not just the physical aspects of a condition, but the entirety of an individual's life. In doing so, we pave the way for a healthcare system that truly sees, understands, and empowers every person it serves.

In envisioning the future of paediatric healthcare, my hope is that the younger generation embarks on their healthcare journey with a profound sense of wholeness. This entails recognizing and harnessing their inherent skills and resources, thus laying the foundation for a transformative transition process. While clinicians often prioritize achieving key milestones during this transition, my emphasis lies in the building and development of *self-autonomy* and a profound sense of *wholeness*.

Embracing wholeness in the context of paediatric healthcare involves viewing each young individual not merely as a patient with specific medical needs, but as a complete and unique person. It means acknowledging the intrinsic skills and resources that reside within them, beyond the spectrum of their medical condition. This holistic approach reframes the narrative, shifting the focus from a set of milestones to the cultivation of self-advocacy, communication skills, and the ability to navigate the goal-setting process.

The transition from paediatric to adult healthcare is a critical juncture that shapes the trajectory of a young person's life. Traditionally, the emphasis during this period has been on achieving specific milestones, marking the completion of one stage and the initiation of another. However, my hope is to redirect attention towards the qualitative aspects of this transition, placing significant importance on the development of self-autonomy.

When an individual has embraced their wholeness, they are equipped with the tools to become effective self-advocates. This includes the ability to engage in meaningful conversations with healthcare providers, articulate concerns, and actively participate in the goal-setting process. It's not merely about reaching the next phase, but about doing so with a profound understanding of oneself and the capacity to actively shape one's healthcare journey.

Solution-Focused Principles

To facilitate this transformative approach, the integration of solution-focused principles within paediatric healthcare spaces becomes crucial. Applying this framework to the paediatric healthcare transition allows clinicians to guide young individuals towards realizing their "whole" selves. Solution-focused principles inherently emphasize the client's autonomy, focusing on solutions rather than problems. Integrating these principles into healthcare spaces creates an environment where young individuals are encouraged to explore their strengths, articulate their aspirations, and actively participate in decision-making processes related to their health.

In envisioning paediatric healthcare spaces that champion solution-focused principles, the emphasis is on creating a *collaborative and empowering* environment. Clinicians become facilitators in the journey of self-discovery, encouraging young individuals to express their interests, preferences, and concerns beyond the clinical realm. These healthcare spaces become platforms where self-advocacy is not only encouraged, but cultivated. By adopting solution-focused practices, clinicians can guide youth in exploring their inherent skills and resources, helping them recognize their capacity for growth and development throughout the transition process.

As we look towards the future of paediatric healthcare, it is a call for *transformation* – a shift from a milestone-centric approach to one centred on the development of self-autonomy and wholeness. The integration of solution-focused principles offers a roadmap for this transformation, creating spaces where youth are not just patients, but active participants in their healthcare journey.

Conclusion

My hope for the youth navigating the paediatric healthcare system is rooted in the belief that embracing wholeness will redefine their transition journey. By recognizing their inherent skills and resources and fostering solution-focused healthcare spaces, we empower young individuals to become not just recipients of care, but architects of their own well-being. The path to a "whole" self is illuminated by a healthcare system that values autonomy, self-advocacy, and the unique potential within each young person.

12 The Power of Compassion and Gratitude

Gunjan Seth

I am a mother of an amazing, lovely boy with autism, ADHD, and unique abilities. My son inspires me with his immense love for everyone. I am also a proud immigrant and very thankful for the land I live on. For me, every moment starts with deep compassion, authenticity, and gratitude. Before exploring Solution-Focused Health Care Coaching (SFHCC) and becoming a certified Solution-Focused Health Care Coach, I failed to notice how much there was to be thankful for, and the miracles happening every day.

As an immigrant to Canada, my family and I faced immense barriers and struggles as newcomers in this country. Those struggles were amplified during my journey as a caregiver for my son. Navigating and advocating for his needs in various, unfamiliar systems has been so hard and this process impacted my mental health, emotional health, and physical well-being. I felt broken, lost, and unable to see or appreciate the many beautiful moments, blessings, and gifts around me.

Since childhood, I have always had a deep passion and hunger to learn, and my hunger to learn increased deeply after my son received his diagnosis. I have always been curious to learn and explore different interventions and tools that might help us both to grow and thrive in the system. However, it was not an easy journey and there were many challenges and learnings for us both.

Initially, I was simply curious about SFHCC. To be honest, I was not even very sure about my ability to participate in such a program. I felt that my participation would be negatively impacted by language and cultural barriers, and that these barriers would be amplified in a model that focuses on communication. Yet I felt there was a deep value in what I knew about the model, so I decided to pursue it with deep compassion and commitment. During the initial sessions, I learned about the key values of SFHCC, such as recognizing your own strengths, resources, and supports that are *already* present, and being curious as well as compassionate. These learnings allowed me to self-reflect with self-compassion and helped me to recognize my own strengths and supports available for me in various spaces, including the SFHCC program. Gradually, I started incorporating the learnings from the coaching sessions in various conversations in my

DOI: 10.4324/9781003414490-15

daily life. It became a way of thinking and living. I started walking my talk. I was always looking for moments where I could find the opportunity to simply use a key word or phrase, like: *already, difference,* or *what else*; or to ask a generative question to shine light on my son's unique abilities, and resources so that he could recognize his own strengths and unique talents and to help his service providers also notice his gifts and strengths, allowing him to thrive in the system.

As an example, my son was experiencing worries due to various sounds in his classroom and in order to feel safe he would hide in a corner. SFHCC helped me to shine light on his abilities and to communicate with him in ways that boosted his self-confidence and self-esteem during those moments of distress and worries. With time, SFHCC became so deeply rooted in my conversations that my son with autism started recognizing those key words, and he gradually started using them in his own conversations with me. He is now self-reflecting using various coping and scaling questions to build on his strengths and work towards the goals that are meaningful for him, and that provide him with a feeling of agency and autonomy. Over time, I noticed that the model had become a part of my daily conversations with his teachers, support workers, healthcare workers, clinicians, and many more people I encountered in my daily life. I now use these principles and tools in ways that enrich our lives, while helping to shine a light on his strengths, resources, and supports available to him in his daily life. As a result, my son is more confident and able to work more collaboratively with others. It has given me an incredibly positive perspective and enhanced my confidence to better meet my son's needs.

For parents, advocating for their child's needs in various systems is a continuous process and it requires immense energy. From my own experience, it can be very emotionally exhausting and draining. Advocacy is a very soft and delicate skill that requires deep thinking and observation. SFHCC provided me with various tools to advocate for my son's needs with curiosity, while focusing on strengths, supports, and resources available to him. It has truly changed my outlook towards various complex and challenging situations. I now see moments and every challenging situation with a strengths-based perspective rather than a deficit-based perspective. It is sometimes simply recognizing what is good enough in this moment, and gradually moving towards a preferred future. It is about embracing your vulnerabilities and learning and growing from them.

In addition to advocating for my son's needs, my involvement within the healthcare system has led me to other roles such as Family as Faculty and Family Mentor, where I support and advocate for other families and individuals while always incorporating principles of SFHCC. SFHCC has allowed me to create safe spaces with authenticity, deep compassion, and curiosity for families, future healthcare workers, clinicians, and diverse stakeholders in various spaces. It has allowed me to honour vulnerability without judgement or assumptions. It allowed me to enable other parents who have immense barriers and intersectionalities. See Box 12.1.

Box 12.1   Powerful Impact Example

I had been co-facilitating a newcomer mental health session and many of the participants are immigrant and refugees. Most of them have language, cultural, and accessibility barriers, and they were hoping to experience some belonging. SFHCC helped me to enable those vulnerable participants and create a sense of belonging for them through the use of deep listening, deep observation, and leading from behind with compassion, authenticity, and curiosity.

I feel SFHCC allows me to see every individual as unique, autonomous, and having inherent strengths and resources. It teaches us to be compassionate and lead from behind with curiosity.

During this learning journey, there were skills and tools I found to be particularly helpful:

- Working collaboratively
- The Funnel of Optimal Functioning (identifying where on the funnel a person is and meeting them there)
- Scaling
- Exceptions to the problems
- EARS (Eliciting, Amplifying, Reinforcing, Start again)
- Recognizing inherent strengths and resources
- Noticing differences
- Being curious
- Holding space and deep breathing

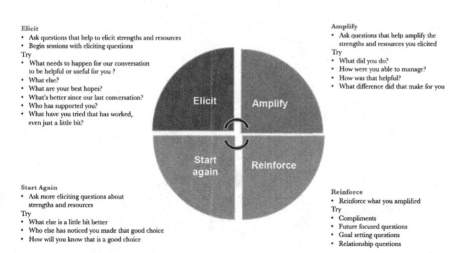

Elicit
- Ask questions that help to elicit strengths and resources
- Begin sessions with eliciting questions

Try
- What needs to happen for our conversation to be helpful or useful for you?
- What else?
- What are your best hopes?
- What's better since our last conversation?
- Who has supported you?
- What have you tried that has worked, even just a little bit?

Amplify
- Ask questions that help amplify the strengths and resources you elicited

Try
- What did you do?
- How were you able to manage?
- How was that helpful?
- What difference did that make for you

Start Again
- Ask more eliciting questions about strengths and resources

Try
- What else is a little bit better
- Who else has noticed you made that good choice
- How will you know that is a good choice

Reinforce
- Reinforce what you amplified

Try
- Compliments
- Future focused questions
- Goal setting questions
- Relationship questions

Figure 12.1 EARS

What connects us with others is our compassion and deep listening. There is a magic in listening deeply with compassion and authenticity, and through the use of SFC I have realized the impact of this magic in various aspects of my life.

I now clearly see miracles happening in our daily lives that I did not even notice in the past. In my role as a Family as Faculty at Holland Bloorview, I am using SFHCC in my conversations with parents, clinicians and, future healthcare workers while co-facilitating various events, and co-teaching students in different settings. My approach to co-facilitation has changed completely. Now, I see myself working collaboratively with clients and families, listening more deeply, acknowledging emotions, creating safe spaces by using clients' language, and leading from behind to meet their hopes. I have been able to grow from someone who was frustrated and exhausted to someone who confidently advocates for my son, myself, and many others, and I have even received awards for Patient and Family Leadership (Children's Healthcare Canada, 2022) and Community Service (from a local community group) for the work that I do with confidence.

Despite the barriers and immense struggles that I have faced, SFHCC has not only enabled me with various tools to support my son and my family, it has also allowed me to develop the confidence to share my new-found skills to shine light on the strengths and abilities of others with similar experiences to my own. It is a very humanistic inclusive approach that breaks down the barriers and leads to a better future for oneself and others.

13 Reflections and Observations as a Parent and Coach of a Child Who Triumphed over Tribulation

Candace Muskat

I have always been interested in the interplay between mental, physical, and spiritual health and the impact these three spheres have on daily living. I'm continually awed by, and curious about, those who experience monumental challenges, yet manage to lead fulfilling lives. What inherent strengths and resources do they tap into, and how do they do it? What enables them to move aside their pain or challenge to notice and make space for the good that exists around them? And what strengthens them to look towards a better future? This curiosity led me to a Master of Social Work (MSW) degree and an early career as a social worker in mental health hospital settings.

Soon after completing my degree, I became that person faced with a monumental challenge. My child fell into a coma due to a serious illness. I entered every parent's worst nightmare. We spent two months in hospital on a knife's edge. Although he miraculously emerged, our robust, active child had been replaced by a mere version of himself, confined to a reclining wheelchair, unable to hold himself up straight, with wide sweeping involuntary movements, poor speech, and significant hearing loss. The sight of him brought me to tears. This new reality was startling. In what seemed like an instant, my active, articulate, happy-go-lucky child could no longer do any tasks of daily living on his own, which meant that we transitioned to the world of paediatric rehabilitation for the next part of this journey.

The intake process for my son's outpatient rehabilitation program all those many years ago is still etched in my mind, and not in a good way. The intake nurse greeted me with the infamous "*what are your goals*" question. I was dumbfounded. Goals? What goals would those be? We had just barely survived two months in hospital; I was exhausted, overwhelmed, bewildered, scared, and confused. At that moment, I didn't even know what a goal was, never mind what I should expect of myself or my child. I responded that my only goal was to drag myself out of bed, brush my hair, get dressed, get my two little girls to school, and make it to the rehabilitation program with my son by 9 am. Without looking up from her notes, the nurse wrote it all down, without any acknowledgement or compassion. Then she went on to say, without missing a beat, or looking up, that given the seriousness of my son's previous illness and the subsequent recovery plan, I might want to book an appointment with the neurologist to learn about the

DOI: 10.4324/9781003414490-16

brain and brain injury. I couldn't believe what I was hearing. This was the first time I heard the term *brain injury*. My small reserve of hope was dashed. By the time the conversation and intake ended, I was in tears, although conversation is a term I would use loosely, knowing what I know now.

The challenge of navigating our complex healthcare system became personal very quickly. I was being called on to walk the talk. I had so many questions: how would we lead meaningful lives; what resources and strengths do I have as an individual, as a mother, as a marital partner, as a family, and, most importantly, what were the strengths and resources of my child; how can I (we) find the positive when everyone around us is focused on the problem(s); who and what will support us; how was I going to ensure that this child was going to grow up to become his best self. It was an abstract journey with no end in sight framed by our shock, disorientation, confusion, and despair. Every day, I wondered: will anything ever be good enough and how will I know?

Eight years ago, I came back to the hospital where my son was a rehabilitation client for 8 months. I was eager to "give back" and share with other parents what I thought they needed to know about navigating our healthcare system, to give hope to and empower others through my story. I considered myself an expert with much to teach.

I became a volunteer Family Mentor with lived experience at the Family Resource Centre of Holland Bloorview Kids Rehabilitation Hospital. I quickly discovered that although I may have expertise in healthcare navigation and resources, I was no expert of anyone else's healthcare journey. Instead of sage advice, most parents and caregivers simply wanted help filling out daunting mountains of endless paperwork. Yet, minutes into the conversation, I would learn that what they really needed was an opportunity to talk about the demands of raising a child with a significant challenge. They had lots to unload. After attending to their stories with deep attention, I'd ask simple questions and offer gentle compliments such as: Wow, how did you manage to get here with your toddler and a baby in a stroller in such weather; or, I'm so impressed that you made it today, given all the stresses. These strategies opened doors to conversations they desperately wanted to have about how they had been managing. These simple questions helped to build rapport and amplified their strengths. It became obvious that when individuals notice their own inherent strengths and resources, they feel empowered to face what seemed too difficult, and even a lengthy financial assistance form can begin to look much less intimidating.

These simple questions and compliments were skills associated with the solution-focused approach to which I had been introduced as part of my social work education and training. I found myself using some concepts intuitively, especially during my son's rehabilitation. So, when I learned about the opportunity to enroll in the Certified Solution-Focused Health Care Coaching (CSF-HCC) year-long program, I was certain it would enhance my skills as a family mentor; however I was completely unaware of the impact it would have on my personal life as well.

I embarked on the certificate program in an effort to refresh what I thought I already knew and to dust off some theoretical concepts, as well as learn the necessary coaching skills and language to enhance my role as a family mentor. I needed more than intuition, I needed to be strategic if I really wanted to offer the best care possible. The skills I developed in that year were nothing short of life-changing.

This year-long program offered many moments of great insight for me as I worked to integrate what I was learning into practice. Being able to be a part of others' ah-ha moments was both humbling and rewarding. The well-designed and integrated formal classes, coaching sessions in front of peers, and the ongoing supervision provided in-depth learning, practice, and nurturing, which formed a foundation for expanding curiosity and discovery.

Although I found the learning broad, exciting, challenging, and deeply gratifying, I often felt as if I was learning a new language. I sometimes felt stuck as I concentrated deeply on substituting new words for those I recognized as no longer valuable in collaborative conversations. I learned to change "active listener" (an old favourite social work term) to being present, and "empowerment" to amplifying and reinforcing. I noticed ways in which I could diminish my own "expertise" as awareness of the wholeness of others developed. I loosened my desire to "fix." I learned how words and language become the vehicles to change our brains, our culture, and our institutions. All of it was powerful and gave rise to a new way of thinking for me. I began to substitute "when" for "if" and "and" for "but." I noticed how even the smallest words matter. This is not just a lesson title, it's a precursor to any form of communication. This simple and challenging new language fostered a new mindset. I was learning to develop positive assumptions that strategically helped clients move from the "if" to the "when." These words were rooted in a world of possibility, potential, and change. The humanistic lens that permeates the entire program shines a light on people as whole and not broken, with unique strengths and resources waiting to be uncovered. If this was all I had learned, I could have said it was good enough because it impacted me so greatly. But there was more.

Along with a shift in vocabulary came a shift in noticing the good and the small wonders in daily life. I challenged myself to reframe just about everything and anything, which helped me practise *leading with a positive assumption* in conversations. For example, a child badgering a parent for another cookie was wonderfully tenacious instead of annoying. A child who did poorly on a presentation has an opportunity to improve and grow from the experience. I became better at shifting the focus from problem-oriented to possibility-oriented. Reframing everyday mishaps and bumps speaks to the solution-focused concept of having one foot in the door of acknowledgement and one foot in the door of possibility. Learning to hold this tension helped me to keep my attention – even in the midst of a challenging conversation – on the client's strengths and resources where the means for a better future exists. See Box 13.1.

Box 13.1   The Gift of Good Enough

We noticed, through our extensive work with clinicians and parents, that both were, and are, often overwhelmed by the constraints of the healthcare system and the work of caring for a child with complex needs. We introduced the concept of "good enough" to help relieve those emotional burdens. Asking a parent or staff member, for example: *"What might be good enough in this moment, given everything else that is going on?"* We constrain the question with time, "in this moment," as well as how it is situated in their life/work context, "given everything else that is going on." These constraints help the individual to know that good enough isn't forever, it is at this point in time. Good enough works beautifully as part of a scaling question, coping questions, and even the miracle question. Individuals are so relieved by the idea that what they are already doing might be good enough, that many become emotional and report that that question alone has been transformative for them.

A strategic question is a coach's best tool and I quickly learned that, to develop the skill of asking well-placed questions, much is required. A solution-focused conversation is strategic and dialogic. The role of the coach is to ask strategic questions that open the right doors for the client to move through, propelling them closer to that which they are seeking to find. When the coach is focused solely on formulating the next great question, it becomes impossible to be present, which critically undermines the dialogic nature of a solution-focused conversation. This was one of my greatest learning challenges. I wanted to ask great questions while being fully present. I began to approach conversations with three messages to myself: (1) Don't interrupt; (2) Don't give advice; and (3) Honour silence. When I was able to follow these three self-prescribed rules, something magical happened: my genuine curiosity gave rise to authentic, beautiful, and strategic questions!

To really integrate theory into practice, a coach needs to find as many coaching opportunities as possible so that new skills can be practised. The informal learning classes embedded in our curriculum were devoted to coaching. During these classes, we could observe and learn from others, develop comfort, proficiency, and our own style in using the skills being taught. Aside from the monthly informal learning sessions where we coached in a group setting and had the benefit of feedback from our co-coaches, it was vitally necessary to seek opportunities to coach friends, family members, and colleagues. I became adept at turning casual phone conversations into coaching opportunities. Even a 5-minute conversation with a stranger became an opportunity to elicit, amplify, and reinforce. And in so doing, I became even more aware of the beauty of humanistic interactions and the ripple effects of respecting others' wholeness, agency, and autonomy. My greatest challenge and achievement over the year was allowing myself to be vulnerable in order to fully experience what was being taught. Exposing my coaching skills to the observations of peers, coaching with co-coaches, and learning from those with greater experience enabled me to develop and grow, as well as become more respectful and appreciative of diversity and commonality.

Solution-focused questions aren't just reserved for coaching clients, work colleagues, or my family. I ask myself these questions in situations where I'm confused, overwhelmed, ruminating, or simply seeking clarity. Questioning myself has become a useful tool.

My reflections on the difference this year of learning made both professionally and personally are profound. In the broadest sense, I feel more free. The more I am able to ground myself in the belief that each individual has their own agency and autonomy, I feel less inclined to try and solve their dilemmas, offer my advice, and fix what wasn't even broken in the first place. I judge less, while noticing and appreciating more. My best hope is that this freedom makes space for others to notice and find their own inherent strengths and resources. As I learned the skills of amplifying and reinforcing, I play a better role in helping others to actualize their best selves.

My family were the first to notice when I started to back off from giving advice and trying to fix everything. It surprised me that instead of embracing this change, it frustrated them. They were accustomed to my quick advice, suggestions, and opinions, especially when they needed to resolve something urgent. The change in my approach, although unwelcomed at first, has been one of my best parenting insights. What tells me that? When I respond with questions instead of answers, I'm hearing less of "please don't use that solution-focused stuff on me" and more of "thanks, that was actually helpful." I can see clearly that questions that stem from my genuine curiosity are much more helpful and supportive because the questions shine a light on their strengths and potential which is what is required to solve their own problem. I also notice that my questions are more genuine and sincere because I'm listening more to understand instead of listening to correct or challenge. I knew something significant shifted when my daughter told a sibling "mom just coached me and she's actually pretty good."

Admittedly, my attention and focus are now firmly grounded in strengths and resources; however, when my child became a rehabilitation client, I was surprised even way back then to discover the profound focus on problem(s) and numerous predictions about the limitations or the possible ramifications of his illness (because he didn't have a diagnosis at the time). As parents, we worked hard to find the positives, looking for new ways for our son to achieve his goals and dreams; however, practitioners worried that our enthusiasm for trying new things would end with disappointments and feelings of failure for our child. His team labelled our goals as risky, while we felt they were far too reserved. For example, when we noticed that our son wasn't compliant with physiotherapy exercises because he felt they were childish and boring, we reframed the process and called physiotherapy "snowboarding strengthening exercises." We knew his dream was to learn to snowboard prior to his illness and so we asked for his rehabilitation to be geared towards strengthening his body in ways that would support that goal. We even gave the therapists suggestions to help them reframe the therapy for our son's success.

We asked them to use snowboarding as a carrot, to shift their language. In no time at all, he couldn't get enough of these snowboarding exercises. However, when the physiotherapist learned that we promised him a snowboard, we were invited to an *emergency round* (his entire care team and my husband and I crammed into a small room), where we were told that we were setting him up for failure. We told the team that his snowboard would hang on his bedroom wall until he's ready. Meeting over.

My son, who is an author, a social worker, and a teacher, describes our frustration best when he wrote in an article:

> What was missing from those hospital and subsequent rehab conversations all those years ago were words that cultivate a growth mindset and discussions about aspirations, possibilities, and solutions … One of the greatest gifts my parents ever bestowed upon me was the mindset of never giving into my challenges or giving up on my potential, and how great I could be despite everything and everyone who seemed to suggest otherwise. The choice was solely up to me – to see obstacles or to see opportunities.

An eight-and-a-half-year-old got it, in spite of the adult clinicians around him.

When a person's wholeness, agency, and autonomy are respected and valued, there is no limit to what can happen. In SF coaching, the client is regarded as being in charge of their own healthcare journey. Coaches support that journey by helping to elicit the client's strengths and resources, and even if the goal isn't met, there is often greater satisfaction in the journey.

By putting the client and their family in the driver seat of their own healthcare journey, healthcare providers can begin to understand what it is their clients want instead of the problem they are currently facing. A future focus better equips clients to find solutions that are meaningful to them. Embracing and celebrating all people just as they are, and supporting what they want by shifting the focus from problem to solution, the future of healthcare can be reshaped for the better. In our case, we weren't asking the clinicians to withhold their expertise – we were asking them to grant our son and our family the space to amplify and reinforce strengths that were already present, and to see where that leads. Rehabilitation is a life-changing journey, and when clinicians respect and support their clients' agency and autonomy, the outcome can be (surprisingly) wonderful. For my son, that snowboard never hung on the wall – it's been on his feet since the age of 9. He's not a good snowboarder, he's an excellent one.

At intake 25 years ago, my child could not hold his body up straight and the sight of him made me cry. Today, I see a tenacious, determined, athletic, and vibrant young man who has learned to become the author of his own life journey as he continues to expand his agency and autonomy, forever reaching higher and finding new potential and possibilities. To use his words, "the choice was solely up to me – to see obstacles or to see opportunities." As a certified solution-focused healthcare coach, I understand that statement more now than ever.

With one foot in the door of acknowledgement and one foot in the door of possibilities, one never knows how the journey can unfold and where it will lead.

Reframing Our Experience

I can best share my favourite solution-focused healthcare coaching skills by contrasting my son's intake experience with what I know now as a certified solution-focused healthcare coach. The following is how I can now re-write that first intake experience so others have the opportunity to become the authors and authority of their own healthcare journey.

Instead of beginning the conversation with a broad general question, such as what are your goals, start *building rapport* immediately by acknowledging where a person is at. *Listen deeply* to what a client is telling you and let them know you've heard. Using the client's words will help to achieve this. *Amplify* and *reinforce* what has already taken place; this is a strength that the client may not know exists and can draw on in the future. A better approach looks something like:

> *Wow, it's been a tough few months for you, and yet you managed to drag yourself out of bed, brush your hair, get your two little girls to school, and show up by 9! What a feat! Would it be helpful to know what you can expect over the next few months?*

Building rapport from the outset is the foundation to building trust and respect. This needs to continue from beginning to end in all conversations. The use of the *EARS model*, eliciting, amplifying, reinforcing strengths, then starting again, facilitates the sharing of information that can be positively highlighted. *Notice* where a client is emotionally and *go slow*, especially when someone presents in a state of despair. It's crucial to get familiar with the *behaviour funnel* (*funnel of optimal functioning*) which will help in determining what type of questions to ask or when to simply hold space. I was so low on this funnel that the questions and suggestions only added to my confusion and I left the conversation in a worse state. Show compassion and let the client know you care about their unique situation and what's important to them. This can be illustrated in the following way:

> *We're going to invite you to come to family rounds to learn more about your son's rehabilitation program. What's one thing that might be helpful for the team to know that I could share on your behalf? Or, What's one thing we should start working on with ... (use the child's name!) right away?*

Get on the same page as the caregiver and *lead with constraints*. As enthusiastic as clinicians may be to share every resource and strategy, the conversation can be constrained in a multitude of ways. For example:

> *What's something you would find useful to know or do today? Would that be good enough for now?*

Understand what's good enough for now. There will be plenty of time to suggest resources and to educate and to expand the plan. By leading with constraints, we can help clients figure out what's *good enough* for small increments of time, so things stay manageable and goals become attainable. To offer the big picture up front is meaningless when we know constraints change, goals change, and strengths and resources build. Small steps can take us to big changes. I know this because although my son is left with a significant hearing loss as well as the loss of two digits on his right dominant hand, he is no longer the child I took to that first intake interview for rehabilitation.

Section Four

Leadership

14 A Humanistic, Solution-Focused Approach

Implications for the Legal System

*Anna Trbovich**

I am the mother of a child with a disability and a lawyer in the criminal justice system. In my life, these two roles usually clash. But there is one way in which these two roles mesh in a surprising and wonderful way: solution-focused coaching. As I will explain in this chapter, I came to learn about solution-focused coaching through my family's association with a paediatric rehabilitation hospital, and it has had a remarkable impact on me as a mum and as a lawyer. In fact, I am now in the process of becoming a certified solution-focused coach. Learning about solution-focused coaching has also inspired me to dream about the difference a solution-focused approach could make in the legal system as I experience it. In this chapter, I will discuss my journey towards pursuing my certification as a solution-focused coach, and I will offer my ideas about how the legal system could benefit from incorporating a solution-focused approach to communication. My journey starts with who I am as a person and as a parent.

Who Am I?

I am the mother of two amazing boys, K and R. K has cerebral palsy and a number of other disabilities and medical issues. He requires assistance with all activities of daily living. K cannot walk, talk, sit, or eat independently. But that doesn't really describe him. Let me try again.

K is a hoot and a half. He deeply and viscerally adores music. In particular, he has had a life-long love affair with Anne Murray's album *There's a Hippo in My Tub*. He also gets massively excited whenever I sing one of my silly old summer camp songs that remain stuck in my brain from my childhood. In addition to Anne Murray and the silly summer camp song genre, K loves the much-missed John Prine and Gordon Lightfoot. The breadth of his music taste is quite something.

K also has a hilarious, contagious, snorty laugh. He loves receiving and giving kisses. He has a big brother who would climb mountains for him. He has a family that loves him more than they can properly put into words. He has a caregiver who calls him her "special love boy." Simply put, he is surrounded by love.

Being K and R's mum is the most important role in my life. And, as I noted at the beginning of this chapter, it often clashes with another important role I have – being a lawyer. I became a lawyer almost 20 years ago. I spent the first decade of

DOI: 10.4324/9781003414490-18

my career as a criminal prosecutor. I worked on adult and youth prosecutions. The crimes I prosecuted ranged from minor thefts to murder. In my second decade as a lawyer, I have been working as a staff lawyer for an appellate court. As a staff lawyer, I am no longer in the courtroom; instead, I am behind the scenes, supporting the work of judges and court administration staff.

I changed my job in large part because I could not manage being a prosecutor and also being K's mum. I could not manage running trials while also running to the doctor, the physiotherapist, the orthotist, the seating clinic, the feeding clinic, the speech and language clinic, etc. I also could not manage dropping everything work-related whenever K had a breathing emergency and was admitted to the hospital. Something had to give, and it was my career.

How Did I Come to the Holland Bloorview Humanistic Health Care Coaching Certificating Program?

It was not easy for me to put my legal career in the back seat. I was an overachiever in school. I graduated first in my high school, undergraduate, and law school classes. I was a law clerk at the Supreme Court of Canada. I did a master's degree in law at Harvard on a full scholarship. In a warped sort of way, as a result of these successive achievements, I felt like I "deserved" success going forward. I didn't. I thought I was invincible. I wasn't. I was convinced I could accomplish anything if I just tried hard enough. I couldn't.

In 2017, I was diagnosed with clinical depression. I took a mental health leave from my job as a prosecutor. During that leave, I made the decision to change my job. I also decided to commit myself to improving my mental health. I attended regular psychotherapy sessions. And, in time, I came to learn about life coaching.

Before I had any personal experience with life coaching, I really didn't know much about it. My casual understanding of it just came from stereotypes I had somehow absorbed from the media and others. For example, I worried it might be something that was just for wealthy people or that it might be a bit of a scam. Was I ever wrong!

My first actual exposure to life coaching was via the podcast *The Lawyer Stress Solution*, which eventually transformed into the *UnF*ck Your Brain* podcast. And it truly did what it says to my brain! The host of the podcast is a lawyer-turned-life-coach named Kara Loewentheil. Ms Loewentheil is a graduate of Harvard Law School. Her coaching focuses on creating a feminist mindset revolution. I saw a little bit of myself in her and this helped me to challenge the stereotypes I had in my mind about life coaching. I found Ms Loewentheil's podcast to be very helpful with my struggles as a lawyer, as a mum, and generally as a human being. So helpful, in fact, that I joined "The Clutch," her online feminist coaching community. It was there that I learned the true impact of one-on-one coaching. And that inspired me to hire a coach of my very own, Tricia Bolton (also a lawyer), so I could take my mindset work even deeper.

This type of coaching has been a game-changer for me. Put simply, my brain works differently now because of it. Importantly, I better understand the impact of my thoughts – both unintentional and intentional – on my feelings and actions. Because of this, I work smarter, rest easier, and love harder. I am very grateful for this development in my life.

Once my mental health leave was over, I started in my new role as a staff lawyer at the appellate court. I also decided to volunteer as a Family Leader at Holland Bloorview Kids Rehabilitation Hospital.

Holland Bloorview is an incredibly important part of my son K's life. His developmental paediatrician is at Holland Bloorview. He is connected to a physiotherapist and an occupational therapist there, as well as the communication and writing aids team. He visits the Feeding Clinic and the Seating Clinic. As a family, we enjoy swimming in the accessible pool there. Sometimes, I feel like our wheelchair van knows the way to Holland Bloorview by itself!

Given the many opportunities and support that Holland Bloorview has given K over the years, I had always wanted to volunteer there and give back. In my new job, I felt like I had the space – mentally and time-wise – to finally do it.

As a Family Leader, I have had the good fortune to support the hospital in all sorts of initiatives, from presenting about client- and family-centred care at new staff orientation sessions to providing feedback on information pamphlets. Family Leaders are also informed about the various programs available at the hospital for staff and volunteers. When I saw that Family Leaders were invited to apply to the Holland Bloorview (HB) Humanistic Health Care Coaching Certification program in the fall of 2022, I was really intrigued, given the positive experience I had with life coaching generally. I knew some Family Leaders who had gone through the program before, but I didn't really know what it would entail.

I did some research and learned that the program's emphasis would be on developing participants' solution-focused communication and coaching skills within the healthcare context and through a humanistic lens. I also learned that the program would be a combination of formal learning, practice coaching, and peer supervision. And I learned that the program was accredited by the Canadian Council of Professional Certification. All of this sounded amazing to me, and I jumped at the opportunity.

My Experience in the Holland Bloorview Humanistic Health Care Coaching Certification Program

At the time I am writing this, I am three-quarters of the way through the Holland Bloorview Humanistic Health Care Coaching Certification Program. The program has been both a "mind-expander" and a "skill-developer" for me.

My mind has been expanded by the program's formal learning component. I have not been in the position of a student in a formal learning environment for quite some time, and I am really energized by this opportunity. Every session, I learn something new (and write down at least one book recommendation), but I also witness and absorb the teaching style of my instructor, Dr Elaine Cook. In each formal learning session, Elaine is not just teaching the new, topical information to us, she is also gently encouraging us to voice our views and insights as well as showing us – by actually doing it in class – how to apply a humanistic and solution-focused lens to teaching. This may sound "clunky," but it is actually seamless and wonderful to experience.

My skills as a solution-focused coach have really developed in this program, both through my practice coaching sessions and through the supervisor meetings where we analyze parts of those sessions. At the beginning of the program, I felt quite nervous doing the practice coaching and I would often have trouble really listening to the person I was coaching, mainly because I would be trying to think of my next question and panicking about this. This was quite akin to my experience as a new prosecutor and conducting an examination-in-chief. This makes sense, because a coaching conversation and an examination-in-chief are, at their essence, examples of strategic dialogue. As I gained experience as a coach, just like when I gained experience as a prosecutor, I learned that my next question would come more easily and naturally when I quieted my mind and focused on listening to what the coachee/witness was saying. I learned that a dialogue cannot happen properly without careful listening.

As I progress through this training program, I am also learning to be thoughtful and strategic about the type of questions I ask and when I ask them. One of the basic aims of a solution-focused coach is to ask *generative questions* to help elicit, amplify, and reinforce the coachee's own strengths and resources, but there are many different types of these questions – for example, *relationship questions* ("What might [a very important person to you] say the difference might be when you are doing X?"), *scaling questions* ("On a scale of 10 to 0, where 10 is high and 0 is the opposite, where would you say you are with respect to X goal?"), *coping questions* ("How did you manage to do that?"), *exception questions* ("When the problem was just a little less, what was different?"), etc. – and the careful timing of their deployment can really propel a session forward.

In order to learn about when to use a particular question, in the course of this training program, I have been introduced to the Funnel of Optimal Functioning (FOF). This is a model that helps coaches determine which solution-focused coaching skills, including but not limited to the generative questions discussed above, to use in a particular session in order to best serve a client's needs (Cook, 2022). When a client is at the bottom of the funnel, their limbic or emotional brain is in control and we may notice them acting stressed, anxious, depressed, etc. (Cook, 2022). The FOF model tells us that now is not the time to give the client information or pepper them with thought-provoking questions; rather, the strategy to use in these circumstances is *holding space* (Cook, 2022). We hold space by reducing stimuli, slowing down our speech, and leading with constraints, for example, "Given that your work schedule was out of your control this week, how were you able to still get that task done?" (Cook, 2022). Conversely, when a client is at the top of the funnel, their pre-frontal cortex is online and they are positively engaged in the session. In these circumstances, the FOF model tells us that this is the time to *elicit, amplify, and reinforce* strengths and resources using generative questions (Cook, 2022).

As a new coach, the FOF model helped me to tailor my practice coaching sessions to where the client was at at that particular time. Without the FOF model, I think I would have been more likely to fall back on the same general set of questions for each practice session no matter what the circumstances. The FOF model encouraged me to move away from this and to really try to notice the client's behaviours in the session and think strategically about how best to support them. Thinking about a client in terms of where they were on the funnel in a visual sense also gave me a benchmark of sorts. As a coach, I wanted to ensure my support did not drive the client any further down the funnel and, ideally, I wanted to see if, through the coaching intervention, they moved up the funnel at all. Overall, I have found the FOF model to be one of the most significant tools for developing my skills as a solution-focused coach.

How the HB Humanistic Health Care Coaching Certification Program Has Made a Difference in My Life

In addition to functioning as a "mind-expander" and a "skill-developer," the HB Humanistic Health Care Coaching Certification Program has made a remarkable difference in my life as a mother of a child with disabilities and as a lawyer.

The Difference the Program Has Made in My Life as a Mother of a Child with Disabilities

I am a happier and more loving mother as a result of taking the HB Humanistic Health Care Coaching Certification Program. In the program, I am continually reminded that each person is already whole. I have taken this lesson to heart. I am whole. My child is whole. This looks easy to write and easy to say, but it is monumental to mean it. Day in and day out, the healthcare system, the education system, and the social services system tell me – scream at me – that my child is broken. I am broken. My family is broken. We are less because of my son's disability. The humanistic stance of this program has given me the guts to rebel against this poisonous, erroneous message. *We are all whole.* Don't you ever forget it!

As a result of learning about solution-focused coaching, I catastrophize less and look for exceptions more. For example, when K is having leg spasms in the night, I don't automatically go to my well-worn thought pattern that ends in "… and as a result our family will never sleep again and we will all slowly die of exhaustion." Instead, I consider when the spasms are a little bit less and then ponder why that is. I also look for times when the spasms are not there and then I think about how to replicate and perhaps amplify those conditions. And, even if I can't replicate or amplify those conditions, or even if the spasms happen despite those conditions being in place, I have learned to acknowledge and derive some comfort from the simple but powerful fact that there are times when the spasms do not happen.

I also wonder what our family's life in the Neonatal Intensive Care Unit (NICU) would have been like if we had had access to solution-focused coaching. K spent two months in the NICU, and he generally cried whenever he was awake and not feeding (due to some kind of neuro-irritability, we think). It was horrible. It nearly broke me. It nearly broke my husband. I think it nearly broke some of the NICU nurses! I remember when we were preparing to leave the NICU, I couldn't imagine how we were going to cope with the crying at home. I was so worried that, in a weird way, I actually didn't want to go home. We certainly could have used some solution-focused coaching then. Instead, that period of time when K was pretty much inconsolable, which continued well past his time in the NICU, was one of the most harrowing periods in our lives. Frankly, I am not sure how we survived. I do not want another family to have to endure that. Solution-focused coaching could have made a real difference for us. Maybe it could in the future for others?

The Difference the Program Has Made in My Life as a Lawyer

The HB Humanistic Health Care Coaching Certification Program has made a dramatic impact on me as a lawyer. At the beginning of this chapter, I shared that I changed my job as a lawyer in large part because I could not manage being a prosecutor and also being K's mum. There was another reason too: vicarious trauma.

As a prosecutor, I saw pain and suffering every day, in all justice system participants. And I took it home with me at night. Many times, I couldn't shake the images I saw or the stories I heard that day in court, so I would retreat to my bedroom and ignore my family. I would have nightmares that disturbed me long after I woke up. I'm sure this contributed in part to my eventual diagnosis of depression.

As I progress through the HB Humanistic Health Care Coaching Certification Program, I have been reflecting on my experience as a prosecutor and especially the difference between empathy and compassion. I realize now that, as a prosecutor, whether I was in court or in witness[1] preparation, I listened with whole-body empathy, and it really set the stage for the accumulation of vicarious trauma. Listening in the way I did, I saw, heard, felt, and smelled the same things the witness was describing. My brain sort of jumped into theirs and then I couldn't get it out.

As a solution-focused coach, I am learning to listen with compassion instead. When I do this, I accept that the client's story is their own. I am curious about it. I can ask strategic questions about it. I can hold space for it. But it is not my story and I am not them. This approach would have made such a difference for me as a prosecutor.

The Difference a Solution-Focused Approach Could Make in the Legal System as I Experience It

Participating in the HB Humanistic Health Care Coaching Certification Program has also inspired me to reflect on the legal system, as I experience it, and to dream about the difference a solution-focused approach could make in this system. I will share some of my ideas in this section, but before I do so, I wish to be clear that my ideas on this point are different from the concept of problem-solving courts, which are also sometimes referred to as solution-focused courts (King, 2011, p. 1008). These courts typically focus on drug addiction, mental health issues, domestic violence, or other socio-legal problems, and they endeavour to address the underlying human causes of crime and criminal behaviour, often through a therapeutic justice lens (Goldberg, 2011, p. 2). There is no doubt that these types of specialized courts have had a significant impact on the legal system (see, e.g., Bakht, 2005); however, my focus in this section is not on these courts, which are more of a structural response to specific criminal justice issues, but rather on applying a solution-focused approach to communication in ordinary interactions between justice system participants.

These ideas of mine are also different from the idea of using solution-focused brief therapy as a specific tool to support the rehabilitation of offenders within the criminal justice system, both in general (Walker & Hayashi, 2009) and for specific populations, such as young persons (Jordan et al., 2013) and those who commit intimate partner violence (Bolton et al., 2022). When I think about how to incorporate a solution-focused approach in the legal system, I am not thinking about using it to rehabilitate people; I am thinking about using it to rehabilitate how we talk to one another. And, if we can do that – if we can make our interactions and our conversations reflective of our belief that we are all whole and we all have our own strengths and resources – I think we could create some meaningful change.

I also wish to make it clear that my experience in the legal system is limited to the criminal justice system. It is also constrained because: (1) the only role I have ever played in this system is the role of a prosecutor; and (2) I am a white, cisgendered woman. In addition to my ideas about how a solution-focused approach could make a difference in the legal system, I am mindful that there are many others with different viewpoints who would also make wonderful contributions to this discussion. Let's keep it going! Below are my three ideas.

First, I think adding some solution-focused questions to witness preparation sessions before criminal trials could be very empowering for witnesses. When I met with a witness to prepare them to testify, I usually just focused on the basics. After introductions,[2] I would show the witness the courtroom (or a sketch of the courtroom) and explain who sits where and what they do. I would explain the difference between examination-in-chief and cross-examination and also what reply is. I would review some general tips about giving evidence – namely, always tell the truth, listen carefully to the question being asked, ask if you don't understand a word or a question, etc. Finally, I would give the witnesses an opportunity to review the statement they provided to the police earlier in the investigation.

While all of the topics I usually covered in the preparation session are important, they did nothing to address two things witnesses often brought with them to the preparation session and to the trial: performance anxiety (e.g., "I am nervous about speaking about these emotional/private/embarrassing/hurtful/upsetting, etc. issues in front of people") and outcome anxiety (e.g., "I am worried about what the judge will ultimately conclude").

Where witnesses express either or both of these trial-related anxieties (or others), I think some targeted solution-focused questions would really help. The solution-focused questions could be asked by the prosecutor and/or the VWAP staff person, as appropriate. For example, with regard to performance anxiety, the prosecutor or VWAP staff person could ask the witness about what they want to feel *instead of* nervousness when they are testifying and the conversation could build from there, perhaps moving to a set of scaling questions focusing on the goal of feeling X (instead of nervous) and then perhaps moving to some coping questions (e.g., about previous times in their life when they felt nervous and were still able to perform and how they might be able to do some of the same things in this situation). With regard to outcome anxiety, the questions could begin by getting curious about how they want to define success in this situation (i.e., separate from what the judge may ultimately decide). Then, the questions could move to asking what they might notice as the first sign they are moving towards what they defined as success and/or what a very important person in their life might notice as the first sign. In my view, incorporating some solution-focused questions into a witness preparation session could really transform the session. Put simply, these questions could help witnesses step into their own power.

The second idea I have comes from the time I spent as a prosecutor in youth justice court (the court process for those aged 12–17). Often, in cases where a young person has incurred a number of serious charges, the presiding judge will convene a case conference bringing together the young person, their parent(s) or guardian(s), their lawyer, the prosecutor, the police (if appropriate), a probation officer and/or youth justice worker, a representative from the school system (if appropriate), a youth mental health worker (if appropriate), and representatives from other applicable social services. Pursuant to s. 19(2) of Canada's Youth Criminal Justice Act, "[t]he mandate of a conference may be, among other things, to give advice on appropriate extrajudicial measures [in support of diversion], conditions for judicial interim release [bail], sentences, including the review of sentences, and reintegration plans."

While I found these conferences to be very impactful, especially with their expanded focus on the many components of a young person's life, I also found that they still put the court, and more specifically the judge, in the "problem-solver" role rather than in the role of "facilitator" or "supporter" of the young person to generate and implement their own solutions (King, 2011, p. 1008). In fact, in my experience, the young person often did not speak much at these conferences. Instead, much of what was decided at these conferences seemed to "happen to or around" the young person (King, 2011, pp. 1021, 1024).

I think these conferences could become even more impactful if they became more solution-focused – that is, if they became more about what the young person thinks "has helped/is helping/could help" and less about what the adults think "will work" (King, 2011, p. 1031). In my mind's eye, I see conferences dedicated to asking questions of the young person with the aim of helping them become aware of (1) the underlying causes of their offending, (2) their own strengths and resources, (3) how they already may be doing things that are helping to address these underlying causes, (4) how they might do more of what is helping, and (5) what else might be helpful for them in moving towards positive behavioural change and how they might implement it (King, 2011, p. 1022). These conferences would promote the young person's ability to resolve their own problems in the present and, importantly, in the future too (King, 2011, p. 1032). Certainly, the other participants in the conference would still be there to facilitate access to support services and, if necessary, engage in compliance monitoring, and the outcome or decision made at the conference would be negotiated among all participants, with the judge as the ultimate decision-maker (if necessary), but the young person – their wholeness and their self-efficacy – would be at the centre of it all (King, 2011, p. 1033).

The final idea I have has been bubbling in my brain for a while, but it finally broke the surface, so to speak, when I read a recent article in my local paper titled "Addiction. Poverty. Mental Health. Those are the real challenges facing Ontario's justice system, retired judge warns" (Gallant, 2023, 21 May). The author of the article had interviewed a recently retired criminal court judge. This judge had been on the bench for over 30 years and had primarily presided in a busy downtown courthouse whose catchment area included some of the poorest neighbourhoods in the city. The article was unusual, because, where I live, judges – retired or not – rarely give interviews. But this judge wanted to talk in order to "call attention to systemic failures in the justice system."

In the article, the judge observed that there had been "a dramatic shift in the types of cases" handled by her court. Now, accused persons "are not necessarily hardened criminals"; rather, they "appear in court with a history of substance-use disorders, mental health issues, homelessness, or sometimes all three." Accordingly, "the court has had to take on an increase in what some might call 'social work.'" On this point, the judge pithily commented: "To a certain degree, I guess it is social work, but it is our work now."

I agree it is "our work now," and I while I would argue that "our" includes all those who work in the criminal justice system, I think, for many cases, the judge will be best-placed to make the biggest impact on the lives of accused persons facing these "social work" problems. And here is where I think a solution-focused approach could work some magic, just like it has worked some magic in the healthcare sector (see other chapters in this book).

- What if an accused person's appearance in court was an opportunity for them to consider what brought them to court and to engage in some realistic goal-setting in that context?
- What if they were asked about what difference would it make to them when they achieve the goal they have identified?
- What if they were asked about some things they are doing right now that are already moving them towards this goal?
- What if they were asked about previous times when they were successful achieving a goal like this and what would be helpful from back then to leverage now?
- What if, when they returned for another appearance, they were asked about what is a little bit better?

In the article, the judge advocated for judges to get their "annual education on more than just 'hard law,' but on issues that are causing so many people to come before the court." What if, as part of this training, judges were to learn about solution-focused coaching? I think it could lead to profound change.

Conclusion

I never thought I could write something – let alone a chapter in a book – that combined the topics of being a mother to a child with a disability and being a lawyer in the criminal justice system and wasn't just some kind of lament or cautionary tale!

In all honesty, writing this chapter has helped me to appreciate the meaningful impact the HB Humanistic Health Care Coaching Certification Program has had on my life. In her email communications with me and other course participants, Dr Cook often asks, "What did you notice, with glittering eyes, today?" Before I took this course, I didn't even notice I had glittering eyes. Now, I treasure them. With these glittering eyes, I see wonderful things happening in my life as a mum and as a lawyer. I also see amazing possibilities on the horizon for the criminal justice system. This is the gift the program has given to me. This is the gift of a solution-focused approach. I am forever grateful.

Notes

* Throughout my career, I have been a government employee. The views I express here are my own personal ones; they are not the views of my employer. In these pages, I am just me.
1 In this chapter, I am using the general term "witness" to refer to all types of people who end up testifying at a criminal proceeding: complainants, eyewitnesses, expert witnesses, police witnesses, etc.
2 In addition to me and the witness, a police officer (usually the officer-in-charge) would be present at these meetings. Where appropriate, a staff person from the victim witness assistance program (VWAP) would also attend.

References

Bakht, N. (2005). Problem Solving Courts as Agents of Change. *Criminal Law Quarterly*, *50*(3), 224–254.

Bolton, K.W., Hall, J.C., Lehmann, P., Wilkins, M., & Jordan, C. (2022). Strength-based batter intervention programs for intimate partner violence. In C.M. Langton & J.R. Worling (eds), *Facilitating Desistence from Aggression and Crime: Theory, Research, and Strength-Based Practices* (pp. 379–416). John Wiley & Sons Ltd.

Cook, E. (2022). The Funnel of Optimal Functioning: A model of coach education. *The Coaching Psychologist*, *18*(2), 42–57.

Gallant, J. (2023, 21 May). Addiction. Poverty. Mental health. Those are the real challenges facing Ontario's justice system, retired judge warns. *Toronto Star*. Available at: https://www.thestar.com/news/gta/2023/05/21/addiction-poverty-mental-health-those-are-the-real-challenges-facing-ontarios-justice-system-retired-judge-warns.html

Goldberg, S. (2011). *Problem-Solving in Canada's Courtrooms: A Guide to Therapeutic Justice*. National Judicial Institute.

Jordan, C., Lehman, P., Whitehill, K., Huynh, L., Chigbu, K., Schoech, R. et al. (2013). Youthful Offender Diversion Project: YODA. *Best Practices in Mental Health*, *9*(1), 20–30.

King, M.S. (2011). Should problem solving courts be solution-focused courts? *Revista Juridica Universidad de Puerto Rico*, *80*(4), 1005.

Loewentheil, K. (Host). (2017). *The lawyer stress solution* [Audio podcast]. Available at: https://thelawyerstresssolution.com/

Loewentheil, K. (Host). (2017–present). *UnF*ck your brain* [Audio podcast]. Available at:
   https://unfuckyourbrain.com/
Murray, A. (1977). *There's a hippo in my tub* [Album]. Capitol/EMI.
Walker, L. & Hayashi, L. (2009). *Pono Kaulike*: Reducing violence with restorative justice
   and solution-focused approaches. *Federal Probation, 73*(1), 23–27.
Youth Criminal Justice Act, S.C. 2002, c. 1.

15 A Humanistic, Solution-Focused Approach to Meeting the Challenges in Education

Kim Weishar

Introduction: Challenges in the Larger Context

Education and society itself are, as educational researcher Andy Hargreaves describes, "in a crisis like we've never seen before" (Hargreaves, 2024, p. 1). He references what he terms "The Big Five – COVID 19, Climate Change, War, Racism, and Democracy in peril" as setting the context for our current education systems, schools, and classrooms. I would add to this list a few more items – the increasing cost of living, heightened by a significant inflationary period that is affecting the day-to-day living of families as well as an addictions crisis fuelled by the opioid epidemic, which is now leading to a significant increase in the number of students who are being impacted from birth. With constant and easy access to information as well as disinformation, the twenty-first-century education system is heavily impacted by the world in which it orients itself.

The Big Five challenges described by Hargreaves, as well as a soaring cost of living and the destructive prevalence of addiction in our communities, have created a world that feels like it is spinning out of control with regular folks having very little influence to change or transform the conditions that we are living under. Our feelings of agency, safety, and belonging have been significantly impaired by a world that has just emerged from a pandemic and now feels as if it is on the brink of self-destruction.

This lack of agency, safety, and belonging in a fractured world has translated into schools and classrooms that are becoming incredibly challenging to navigate. The education system exists within the context of what is happening in the world surrounding it and the societal impact of the issues of the day. Modern communications have made this world a much smaller place, where instant access to a 24/7 stream of information means that the world enters the classroom every day in many different ways that challenge educators and educational leaders as they attempt to navigate both the positive and negative impact that students, families, and staff experience.

It is a hope and expectation that schools and classrooms will be places of belonging, safety, and achievement, and that has been the case for many students; however, it is not for many others, particularly those who have experienced marginalization due to discriminatory and oppressive practices. Black, Indigenous,

DOI: 10.4324/9781003414490-19

students of colour, LGBTQ2S+ students, and students with disabilities have been clearly telling us for years that schools are not safe or equitable places for them. In their report *Towards Race Equity in Education*, which examined the experience of Black students in Toronto District School Board, published in 2017, Carl James and Tana Turner outline at least 30 years of reports, studies, and commissions that describe the ways that the various provincial governments in Ontario have tried to address the inequitable outcomes for black students. The significant experiences of racism, oppression, discrimination are described again and again with little measurable change towards equity (James & Turner, 2017, p. 6).

The same type of work has been attempted to address the needs of students with special education needs. In 2005, the Ontario Ministry of Education released *Education for All: The Report on the Expert Panel on Literacy and Numeracy Instruction for Students with Special Education Needs Kindergarten to Grade 6* (Ontario Ministry of Education, 2005). This was followed in 2013 with *Learning for All: A Guide to Effective Assessment and Instruction for All Students, Kindergarten to Grade 12*, which was "designed to raise the bar and close the gap in achievement for all students" (Government of Ontario, 2013). In 2022, the Ontario Human Rights Commission released its report, *The Right to Read*, which highlighted inequities in reading instruction faced by students with learning disabilities, as well as Black students, students of colour, and First Nation, Inuit, and Metis students. Despite this ongoing research that amplified the inequities faced by large sections of the student population, school systems continue to seem to be unable or unwilling to address them in any substantial way and schools remain places of safety and belonging for only some students, not all.

However, during COVID-19, schools were shuttered for extended periods of time, and like any public location where people gathered, they became places that were unsafe for everyone. Even when we returned to school, we did so under strict public health guidelines that included masking, social distancing, isolation when showing symptoms of illness, no physical contact, and sitting in rows. Schools looked very different from what we were used to, for both the adults and the children in the buildings. Feeling unsafe in our schools was also exacerbated by COVID-19 where that sense of safety and security in our communities, outside of our homes, was severely compromised. COVID-19 impacted everyone, everywhere in the world, and we were subjected to a constant barrage of images of sickness, death and dying, and the unknown.

Faced with this, how could people not have internalised an overwhelming sense of fear. Rabbi Harold Kushner reminds us that being afraid diminishes our humanity (CBC Radio Tapestry, December 3, 2023). When people are afraid, they are not able to function at their best. This fear is impacting the interactions and encounters that we are seeing in schools – increased violence in the classroom, demands and expectations from parents, and impotence of educators and school leaders to manage and mitigate issues. Students and families who have faced marginalization are rightfully demanding, in no uncertain terms, equitable opportunities, recognition, understanding and consideration of historical trauma and lived experience, and fulsome responses to incidents of racism, discrimination, and harassment both by students and staff. Advocacy groups watched schools change their mode of delivery from face-to-face learning to a virtual environment essentially overnight. The excuse that change in the school system moves slowly was put to rest very quickly as necessitated by COVID-19 public health requirements. Schools, teachers, and students adapted quickly to the virtual environment and, although not perfect, it did demonstrate that the education system could change quickly if necessary.

Challenges in My Context

It is within this global context that I work as part of the senior team as a superintendent of Program Services for a medium-sized Catholic school board in central Ontario with about 24,000 students. We are only about an hour from a major population centre and have seen an influx of families moving to our area because of the housing market. We have also seen a significant increase of newcomers in our communities and schools from around the world, many impacted by war and violence in their home countries. This increasing diversity in our schools is not being matched by diversity in our staff, including leadership at both the school and the senior level: we remain an almost all-White, homogenous group.

In my role, I oversee the implementation of teaching, learning, assessment, and reporting practices, as well as Student Success programs within the context of the Ontario curriculum and the Ministry of Education regulations, policies, and priorities from Kindergarten to Grade 12. This work is supported by a team of 55 teachers and principals who have a wide variety of experience and expertise. As a central team, one of the main things we do is support the professional learning and development of school-based staff, including principals, teachers, designated early childhood educators, and educational assistants, through a variety of models of learning, including large-group face-to-face in-services, small-group professional learning cycles, one-on-one direct support, virtual learning, and resource development and implementation, just to name a few. Our goal is always to be responsive to the needs of the system as well as the individual educators who reach out to us on a day-to-day basis. Most often, the work we do involves interpreting and disseminating curriculum, policy, procedures, and best practices that come from the Ontario Ministry of Education, as well as the latest educational research, into manageable, understandable, and scaffolded chunks that busy educators and leaders can implement effectively in their schools and classrooms. We do this within the context and expectations of equitable and inclusive education principles, as well as culturally relevant and responsive pedagogy.

COVID-19 had put a hold on much of the work the central team was doing to support school staff in the areas of student achievement and well-being and instead led us to focus on health and safety practices and the operations management of our schools. As we and the rest of the world started to slowly emerge from the isolation of the pandemic, we quickly recognized that we were in a much different place than where we had left off. Our staff reported large-scale feelings of burnout and being overwhelmed, exacerbated by daily staffing shortages. There were reports of increased incidences of violence and aggressive behaviour from both students and parents. The academic needs of children after three years of isolation, school closures, and virtual learning were exponential. The demands on our schools and school board to respond to the increased and overwhelming mental health needs in our system was an overarching theme that impacted everyone – staff, students, and families – and as a central team we struggled to support those who served in our schools. As we tried to recreate our pre-COVID-19 schools and classrooms, we recognized that past practices were not going to work. In a space where most people felt safe, and had agency and autonomy, we were able to move the work forward slowly; however, in this new reality of fear, anxiety, and helplessness, we had to do something as a system that would re-establish agency and autonomy and refocus the conversations on possibility, building on the strengths, skills, and resources that we knew our staff and students had.

Anecdotally, staff reported feeling ill-equipped to deal with the complex issues they were facing in schools and classrooms. This was confirmed by our 2021–2022 School Climate Survey Data. In Ontario, all school boards are required by legislation (Ontario Education Act 169.1, 21 & 22) to conduct a Climate Survey at least once every two years. "The purpose of this is to promote a positive school environment and help schools by: assess[ing] perceptions of safety; make[ing] informed planning decisions about programs to help prevent bullying and promote safe and inclusive schools; build[ing] and sustain[ing] a positive school climate" (Ontario Ministry of Education, 2022). A comparison of the data before and after COVID-19 revealed a notable reduction in feelings of engagement, empowerment, and sense of accomplishment.

This change in the data led us to do a deeper exploration of what exactly the impact could be tied to. Overwhelmingly, the increasing complexity of the needs of children in the classroom and the staffing challenges being faced were cited as a factor. Staff felt they were unable to respond to or "fix" the problems students were experiencing, and principals reported feeling unable to manage the day-to-day operations of the school, let alone try to be educational leaders and support the learning agenda. These needs of students were as diverse as the classrooms they were being experienced in, including academic, social, emotional, and psychological needs, as well as the day-to-day physical needs of hunger and safe and stable housing. We were facing daily staffing shortages to the point where classrooms had to be closed for the day due to no available teachers, and students with special education needs had to stay home because of lack of available support staff.

We were seeing a rise in the reporting of violence and racialized situations in the classroom and at school. Parents and advocacy groups of First Nation, Inuit and Metis students, Black students and students of colour, and those who identify as LGBTQ2S+ were highlighting the fact that their educational priorities were not being met in terms of equity, opportunity, representation, and achievement. Staff were expressing feelings of being fearful of doing or saying something wrong, of using what were now considered out-of-date or inappropriate resources that they had traditionally relied on. Educators and leaders described feelings of inadequacy to respond to the diverse needs of students and families because they lacked the lived experience of marginalization and did not have the skills to be able to negotiate difficult conversations they were having with families. There were overwhelming feelings of fear and lack of agency and autonomy to do anything about it.

As senior staff, at the system level, we recognized the importance of a positive school environment where all students, staff, and families felt welcomed, included, and heard. We did specific training and learning ourselves, specifically regarding anti-racism and equity and inclusion. We provided anti-racism and discrimination training to all staff, using the Ontario Human Rights Commission "Call it Out" online training and an internally developed module based on feedback from staff in terms of what they needed to learn more about. Our School Board policies were reviewed and re-written to ensure they reflected current expectations of equity and inclusive education. Significant resources and time were provided to staff to build understanding around issues such as the historical trauma of the residential school system, and the ongoing racism and discrimination experienced by Black students, students of colour, LGBTQ2S+ students, and students with disabilities.

Despite this, staff still reported discomfort and fear as they navigated the complexities of racialized, discriminatory, and oppressive situations. The work we had been doing served to provide context and history, but was failing to provide strategies and skills in how to navigate these complex situations in a way that developed positive relationships and focused on strengths, skills, and resources rather than deficits and problems. We knew what we had to do in terms of providing equitable outcomes for all students; however, we were unsure of how to do it. We felt that our policies and expectations were pretty clear; however, it was also clear that the day-to-day encounters being experienced by students, staff, and families were still being driven by fear, lack of understanding, and perceived power imbalances.

As a system, we needed something that would transform the encounters that staff, students, and families were experiencing within the school system. The training we had been doing to support equity and inclusion was important to set the history and the context, but it was not transformational in how staff, students, and families were experiencing school. We needed to find a way to provide training in principles, skills, and strategies that helped staff navigate complex situations that they were not experts in and where there was not an easy fix or response. We also needed to shift a mindset that included both conscious and unconscious biases, stereotypes, and lack of understanding of the lived experiences of students who faced racist, oppressive, and discriminatory practices in our system. We needed a model that would focus us back on our moral imperative as Catholic educators to recognize the humanity in every person we encountered, and provide learning and work spaces that would support staff and students to flourish.

The Humanistic, Solution-Focused Approach

In the fall of 2022, a small group of our central staff were introduced to the principles, strategies, and skills of Solution-Focused Coaching supported by the framework of the Funnel of Optimal Functioning (Cook, 2022) through a 20-hour mini-certification program. This model was being used successfully in a healthcare setting to support frontline staff in their interactions with clients/patients. The focus on the individual humanity of everyone, and the recognition that people were not broken and came with inherent strengths, skills, and resources, spoke to the team immediately. The supporting evidence of the efficacy of the approach, based in neuroscience, made a great deal of sense to us. It supported other strengths-based educational research that we had been emphasizing for years, such as growth mind-set (Dweck, 2007), grit (Duckworth, 2018), self-regulation (Shanker, 2010), and resilience (Ungar, 2017). We wondered if the same model could be implemented to support system leaders, school leaders, educators, and support staff in their interactions with students, families, and colleagues to promote better understanding of behaviour and emotions and provide skills and strategies that would emphasize strengths, skills, and resources, rather than get caught in a problem-focused dialogue.

To deepen our understanding, skills, and practice of Solution-Focused Coaching, 22 members of a cross-departmental team, including teachers, principals, a speech language pathologist, an assistive technology trainer, a psychologist, mental health staff, and two superintendents, participated in the year-long Solution-Focused Coaching Certification Program. The more we learned, the more we saw the connections and the potential for transforming the way we were supporting the professional growth and learning of our staff and the ripple effect that it might have in our schools and in the classroom. We recognized that this might be the systemic change needed to engage people by acknowledging their current circumstances and reframing the focus on the opportunities that existed to move their encounters with students, families, and colleagues to ones full of hope and possibility.

The Principles of Humanism

One of the most powerful pieces that we have been reinforcing is starting any encounter with an understanding of the principles of Humanism, that everyone comes to us whole, and unique with inherent strengths and resources and a human desire towards self-fulfilment and self-actualization. This principle correlates beautifully with our belief as Catholic educators that every child is formed in the image of God and their dignity is to be valued as a unique being. It supports what is at the core of the purpose of education that Sir Ken Robinson and Kate Robinson describe:

> … all individuals have unique strengths and weaknesses, outlooks and personalities. Students do not come in standard physical shapes, nor do their abilities and personalities. They all have their own aptitudes and dispositions and different ways of understanding things. Education is therefore deeply personal. It is about cultivating the minds and hearts of living people. Engaging them as individuals is at the heart of raising achievement.
>
> (Robinson & Robinson, 2022)

In my own personal practice, starting with this fundamental understanding has changed the way that I engage with those around me. It has allowed me to remain calm in contentious situations and recognize the wholeness of the person in front of me, rather than the brokenness, and then engage in solution-focused conversations that are generative rather than destructive.

The quotation of Dr Rachel Remen, "Wholeness is never lost, only forgotten" (Remen, 2006, p. 108), has resonated with many of us involved in the solution-focused training. The Humanistic principle that students, staff, and families come to us whole, that they are not broken, and that it is not our responsibility to fix them takes an immense amount of pressure away from our role as educators. This has the potential to provide a protective factor for staff. The vast majority of those who work in education do so under the belief that they can make a difference in the life of a child and genuinely want to do what's best for all students in their classrooms and schools. The current context of public education can be overwhelming and heavy to carry, as previously illustrated. Reports of burnout because of not being able to address the many needs have intensified. Recognizing that we are not re-sponsible for fixing the multitude of problems, but instead, engaging with students and families that focus on strengths, skills, and resources has been powerful in changing the negative and helpless narrative that has become so prevalent.

Part of our most current work has been providing professional learning to sup-port the implementation of a new Language and Mathematics curriculum that has been introduced by the Ontario Ministry of Education. My team is in the unenvi-able position of being the messenger of Ministry imperatives that are not always well thought out and appropriately supported. As with many other initiatives that are promoted through a political agenda, there is a great deal of cynicism and sus-picion. The messages we bring are not always well received, as they challenge current practices and potentially create the suggestion that people have been doing something wrong. Remembering that we are not broken, that we are developing and growing as we learn, is a stance that we reinforce with all professional learning we are doing. This has allowed us to focus on moving forward rather than ruminating on what is perceived to be broken with the blame and shame that comes with that.

The Funnel of Optimal Functioning

The Funnel of Optimal Functioning (Cook, 2022) provides a framework for under-standing how people function depending on their emotional state at the time. It then connects that to strategies that can be used to move people up the funnel to better functioning, ranging from simply holding space and breathing with them, to ask-ing questions that elicit strengths, skills, and resources that lead to goal planning and actions. Developing my understanding of optimal functioning and recognizing where I am and where others are on that funnel has been a game-changer in my interactions both at work and in my personal life. It has changed the way that I talk about people who may not be functioning well. Instead of labelling the behaviour as something negative, I am able to focus on where they are on the funnel and what the best strategy might be to help them move up so we are able to engage in posi-tive, solution-focused conversations. I have seen a reduction in escalation of situ-ations and have been able to manage my own emotional responses in challenging interactions. I have also been able to reflect on those situations where I have not managed communication or facilitation well, determined where things went awry, and figured out how I might do better in a similar situation in the future.

Generative Questions

One of the solution-focused aims that we have been developing and focusing on is to *elicit, amplify and reinforce the strengths, skills and resources* that people inherently have and that they should be the authors of their own professional learning journey – we are just the guides. We have done this through utilizing a variety of *generative questions*. Asking good thoughtful questions from a stance of *curiosity and not knowing* rather than simply providing information and expecting change has provided opportunities for conversations that are supporting shifts in mindsets and practices.

We have seen this happen within our own skills as facilitators. In the past, we presented way too much information and would end up overwhelming people who would feel impotent rather than prompting change. Instead, we are now trying to pare down the information to what is essential or most important and allowing time for thought and discussion. We draw on the wisdom of the people in the room to share expertise and experience and have been able to have some very challenging conversations about current practices that are not serving students – conversations we could never have had even a year ago. The questions we use are often very similar and then tailored to the topic, "What are you curious about ...?" "What has worked before? ..." "If you had all the funding, resources, and people, what would the ideal look like?" We have used these questions in both large- and small-group and one-to-one settings and have witnessed the thoughtful shifts that have been happening.

The Best Hopes Question

One of the generative questions that we have implemented in much of our work is the *best hopes question*. This question can be used in a large group, as part of pre-session preparation and post-session follow-up, in one-on-one conversations, and in small-group settings for planning. Members of my team use it to start a session, to set the stage for participants being the agents of their own learning: "What are your best hopes for your learning today?" We also use it to close a session, as part of an exit ticket to measure implementation of new learning and support future planning: "What are your best hopes for the implementation of the learning you have participated in today?" The power of the best hopes question is that it is action-oriented, it suggests that the person has the ability to influence the outcome that they hope for and there are actions they can take to move towards their vision or goal. One of my team members described it beautifully by saying that hoping is different from wishing; wishing does not have action attached to it, the participant is left to the whims of outside influences rather than having the agency and autonomy to have an impact on the outcomes. Hoping allows for actions that move the person closer to their perceived outcome. It allows the participant to focus on their next best step forward, rather than staying stuck in the impossible, thus reinforcing their agency and autonomy.

We are also using the best hopes question on a systemic level by adding it as part of our *Escalation Form*. When a parent, student, staff, or community member has a concern and it is not settled to their satisfaction at the local level, they are able to submit an Escalation Form, which moves it to a senior team member to support resolution. Based on the learning done in the Solution-Focused Coaching Certificate Program, the superintendent with responsibility for this added the question "What are your best hopes in the resolution of this issue?" to the form. We had some concerns that the answers would be the firing of people or other unrealistic objectives; however, that has not been the case. One parent was simply looking for their child to feel safe and happy at school. The answers have given a window into the humanity of the person writing the concern and provided a positive jumping-off point for seeking solutions.

The Scaling Question

The scaling question has also proven to be a valuable tool that we are using in many different situations. From a system perspective, we are using a scaling question ranking from 10 being "the most effective professional learning you have participated in" to 1 being "the least to inform planning and next steps for future sessions." This has given us valuable insight and we are confirming that sessions we do that allow time for processing, thoughtful discussion, and generative questions are more successful and relevant to the participants.

I was recently organizing a session for all of our principals with a Solution-Focused Coaching Facilitator. The facilitator asked me to rank where the principals were on a scale of 10 being "able to best cope with their current circumstances" and 1 being "not able to at all." As a group, I gave them a ranking of 6. This informed our planning, and we provided a session that was helpful and impactful in that moment. I shared with the principals that we had used a scaling question in deciding how to proceed with our session and they confirmed that they were about a 6. It was such a simple tool, yet had a powerful impact.

Conclusion: The Possibilities for Transformation

Participating in the Solution-Focused Certificate Program has reinforced for me and my team that despite referencing strengths-based education for years, the education setting remains very similar to the healthcare one – it is problem-based – when a student is struggling, we look at the symptoms, diagnose the problem, and try to fix it. This problem-focused orientation often leads to negative and demoralizing encounters that a family has with school. It focuses on negative behaviours and learning difficulties instead of building on the strengths and resources that students and families have. It centres the expertise in solving the problem on the educators and the system rather than a collaborative, shared decision-making process. It is clear to us that this is not working for a diverse population of students. It does not engage the student and family as partners and experts in their educational journeys.

Solution-Focused Coaching is helping us to shift this problem-based narrative, by focusing on principles, skills, and strategies that engage students, staff, and parents in conversations that recognize the humanity in each individual we encounter, elicit, amplify, and reinforce the inherent strengths, skills, and resources that people possess, and shift to what people can do rather than what they cannot.

The education system is at a critical juncture that is not going to change through policy or procedures – we have tried that, and have had limited success in transforming to meet the needs of all of our students and families. Transformation is going to happen one conversation at a time and it is critical that educators and leaders recognize and value the equal importance of the lived expertise of the students, staff, and families they encounter and that they have the ability to be agents of their own development and achievement. Solution-Focused Coaching shows us how to do this; it is how we will transform the school system to meet the aspirations of the Universal Declaration of Human Rights that "All human beings are born free and equal in dignity and rights" (United Nations, 1948, p. 4) and that "Education shall be directed to the full development of the human personality and to the strengthening of respect for human rights and fundamental freedoms" (United Nations, 1948, p. 54).

References

Cook, E. (2022). The Funnel of Optimal Functioning: A model of coach education. *The Coaching Psychologist*, 18(2), 42–57.

Dweck, C.S. (2007). *Mindset: The New Psychology of Success*. Random House.

Government of Ontario. (2013). *Learning for All: A Guide to Effective Assessment and Instruction for All Students, Kindergarten to Grade 12*. Available at: https://files.ontario.ca/edu-learning-for-all-2013-en-2022-01-28.pdf

Hargreaves, A. (2024). Leadership paradoxes. In: *Leadership from the Middle* (pp. 17–33). Routledge.

James, C. & Turner, T., with George, R. & Tecle, S. (2017, April). *Towards Race Equity in Education: The Schooling of Black Student in the Greater Toronto Area*. Available at: https://edu.yorku.ca/files/2017/04/Towards-Race-Equity-in-Education-April-2017.pdf

Kushner, H. (December 3, 2023). CBC Radio Tapestry. Available at: https://www.cbc.ca/radio/tapestry/life-enriching-advice-from-harold-kushner-1.5488838

Ontario Human Rights Commission. (2022). *The Right to Read: Inquiry Report. Public inquiry into human rights issues affecting students with reading disabilities*. Available at: https://www3.ohrc.on.ca/sites/default/files/FINAL%20R2R%20REPORT%20DESIGNED%20April%2012.pdf

Ontario Human Rights Commission. (n.d.). Call it Out. Available at: https://www.ohrc.on.ca/en/learning/elearning/call-it-out

Ontario Ministry of Education. (2005). *Education for All: The Report on the Expert Panel on Literacy and Numeracy Instruction for Students with Special Education Needs Kindergarten to Grade 6*. Available at: https://www.oafccd.com/documents/educationforall.pdf

Ontario Ministry of Education. (2022). 2021–2022 School Climate Survey Data. Available at: https://www.ontario.ca/page/promote-positive-school-environment

Remen, R.N. (2006). *Kitchen Table Wisdom: Stories that Heal*. Penguin.

Robinson, K. & Robinson, K. (2022). *Imagine If ...: Creating a Future for Us All*. Penguin.

Ungar, M. (2006). *Strengths-Based Counseling with At-Risk Youth*. Corwin Press.

United Nations. (1948). Universal Declaration of Human Rights. Available at: https://www.un.org/en/about-us/universal-declaration-of-human-rights

16 Humanistic, Solution-Focused Healthcare Leadership

Fostering Psychological Well-Being and Psychological Safety

Amy Hu and Sarah Keenan

Introduction

The most valuable asset in any healthcare organization is its people. At a time when healthcare human resources are a significant constraint, organizations need courageous and humanistic leaders who can lean into the challenges of the current reality *and* create work environments that are psychologically safe and supportive. In this chapter, we describe the urgent state of the healthcare workforce, explore humanistic, solution-focused communication strategies that offer leaders the crucial paradigm shift to lead in this complex healthcare environment, while providing practical tools to move teams forward one step at a time while acknowledging the prevailing challenges in healthcare that offer leaders an opportunity for personal and collective growth – the opportunity to do something different.

To provide a framework (toolbox) for our chapter, we first need an understanding of how psychological well-being (PW) and psychological safety (PS) are defined. PW is one perspective of what is generally known as well-being in psychology circles. The other perspective is known as subjective well-being and often includes attributes like positive affect and a general satisfaction with life (Brown et al., 2020; Lucas et al., 1996). PW is more oriented around humanistic attributes such as self-actualization (Maslow, 1959), autonomy and agency (Nafstad, 2015), and King's (2019) six dimensions of well-being (self-acceptance, purpose, personal growth, positive social relations, mastery, and autonomy). PS is defined as the perception that an environment is safe for interpersonal risk-taking (McClintock & Fainstad, 2022), including the sense of feeling safe to speak up without fear of negative interpersonal consequences (Edmondson, 2018). PW affects job performance (Lin et al., 2022) by influencing motivation, social engagement, behaviour, and emotion (Bayhan Karapinar et al., 2020; Boudrias et al., 2021), while PS has been strongly linked to employee error reporting (which advances safety culture), knowledge-sharing, good decision-making, employee engagement, innovation, and fostering a learning culture (Edmondson, 2018; Grailey et al., 2021; Kingston et al., 2022; MHCC, 2018). Significantly, researchers suggest that positive affect positively mediates both intrinsic and extrinsic motivation, which mediate PW, while PS positively mediates positive affect and PW (Lin et al., 2022).

DOI: 10.4324/9781003414490-20

It seems rather obvious, then, that PW and PS are dimensions of organizational leadership deserving of particular attention. Given the resource and staffing constraints currently plaguing healthcare organizations, psychological health and safety may be essential to improving productivity, retention, and operational success (Shain, 2010). Healthcare leaders are uniquely positioned to influence culture and support staff PW and there is ample evidence that leadership style has a significant impact on workers' mental health and well-being. Some leadership styles – for instance, relationship-oriented, authentic, and transformational – have a positive impact on employees, while destructive and laissez-faire leadership styles have a negative impact on employees' mental health and well-being (Montano et al., 2023). This is just as true in the hierarchical and high-pressure healthcare system (Niinihuhta & Häggman-Laitila, 2022; Umoren et al., 2022), where autocratic leadership may be useful in emergencies, but can have damaging long-term effects on employees' well-being. Change-oriented (O'Donovan & McAuliffe, 2020) humanistic leaders (Wang et al., 2023) play a critical role when it comes to PS (McClintock & Fainstad, 2022) because PS is an interpersonal experience and leaders lead teams. Leaders who can facilitate environments with quality social relationships and communication, collaborative learning, lack of power hierarchies, and the ability to lead from behind model and create PS for their staff (McClintock & Fainstad, 2022).

Current State of Affairs

Healthcare workers have been experiencing stress and burnout in the workplace long before the COVID-19 pandemic, a result of chronic inadequate resources and highly demanding work environments. The pandemic significantly worsened the level of distress experienced by healthcare workers due to factors such as high workload, short staffing, and uncertain working conditions. For example: 96% of healthcare workers reported that their work was impacted by the pandemic and 87% felt more stressed at work during the pandemic (SHCWEP, 2022); 53% of physicians are at risk of burnout and 80% are dissatisfied with their workplace (Canadian Medical Association, 2021); 94% of nurses are experiencing symptoms of burnout (Canadian Federation of Nurses Unions, 2022); and 92% of pharmacy professionals are at risk of burnout (Canadian Pharmacists Association, 2022). While these figures are not exhaustive, they are reflective of the Health Human Resources (HHR) crisis which is now one of the greatest challenges facing the healthcare system today, both nationally and internationally.

The Mental Health Commission of Canada (MHCC) also recognizes that psychological health and well-being is a national priority. The MHCC's National Standard of Canada for Psychological Health and Safety in the Workplace (MHCC, 2018) is a call-to-action for healthcare leaders to actively protect worker mental well-being.

Humanistic, Solution-Focused Leadership

Solution-focused coaching and communication are grounded in principles of humanistic psychology (Cook, 2020). The foundations of humanistic, solution-focused leadership include the fundamental beliefs that people are inherently whole, they have inherent strength and resources and an innate desire to move towards fulfillment (Cook, 2020), and that they are invested in ideas that they themselves generate. Considered a strategic and dialogic model of communication (Bauserman & Rule, 1995), it shifts our understanding of how language and words impact our beliefs about ourselves and the world. These beliefs enable and equip leaders to prioritize the relationships that are at the centre of the healthcare system, as well as foster the possibility mindset that is crucial for system innovation.

Solution-focused leadership requires a subtle yet profound shift in how we see the role of the leader. Although there are times when a command-and-control leadership style may be appropriate, humanistic, solution-focused leadership invites leaders to *lead from behind*, by eliciting, amplifying, and reinforcing the strengths and resources of their staff. The effective humanistic, solution-focused healthcare leader understands when their subject matter expertise is required and when it is not. In fact, the lived-experience expertise of our clients is considered equally valuable to our professional expertise. Outcomes are co-constructed, relationships are emphasized, and possibilities are illuminated. Solution-focused leadership practice fosters relationship-centred healthcare and a culture of safety and learning. All of these principles and strategies are what we identified earlier as leader attributes which positively build PW and PS.

The practice of solution-focused leadership involves the adoption of specific *stances* and *strategies*. In a 2022 article, King and Keenan outlined the connection in clinical interventions between a solution-focused coach's *stances* (defined as beliefs, mindsets, and assumptions), *strategies* (defined as purposefully selected actions or strategies), and their role in supporting client engagement. Using this same framework, we can illustrate the impact of solution-focused leadership on teams and individuals (see Table 16.1). These solution-focused strategies illustrate that leaders can directly influence and nurture many of the factors that promote PW and PS.

There are other advantages for our healthcare systems that humanistic, solution-focused leadership, aside from PW and PS, positively influences. Since the healthcare system is composed primarily of people and their inter-relationships (it is people who receive care, people who provide care, people who run hospitals and institutions, and people who lead teams), the provision of care is neither clinician-centred nor patient-centred; ideally, it is relationship-centred (Suchman et al., 2011). This complex web includes relationships between clinicians, patients, and their families; between inter-professional members of the healthcare team; and between teams and leaders throughout the organization. We already know that the relationship between provider and patient is key to a successful patient outcomes (Jun et al., 2021), and as mentioned above, we know that the well-being of healthcare workers is strongly influenced by their relationship with the individual who leads their team.

Humanistic, solution-focused leadership brings the same partnership, respect, mutual understanding, shared decision-making, and attention to relational processes from the clinical sphere to the employer/employee relationship. Historically,

Table 16.1 Impact of solution-focused leadership

SF leader's stances	SF leader's strategies	Examples	Impact
Leading from behind	Strategic questioning	"I'm curious to know what you appreciated about this event."	Team members feel trusted, listened to; creates opportunities to speak up; nurtures sense of competence, mutual respect; nurtures deeper connection between the leader and the team.
	Use of powerful questions	"When we have achieved our goal, what difference will it make for our patients?"	
	Listening (for what is really important; for what is wanted; for what might be possible)	"What else?" "What difference did that make for you?"	
"AND" mindset; keeping one foot in acknowledgement and the other in possibility	Use of "and" instead of "but"	"You did a great job on this project *and* I need you to make some changes to the presentation." "You are an excellent nurse, *and* you made an error." "This has been really hard on our team *and* we're not giving up."	Moves thinking beyond right/wrong, good/bad; success/failure towards learning, and holding the tension between two seemingly mutually exclusive ideas or polarities. Builds respect, recognition, competence; ability to think creatively.
Possibility mindset	Exploring the preferred future	"What are your best hopes for this project?"	Opens up creative thinking; engages all team members in ownership of team goals; maintains and refocuses on desired outcomes, despite constraints.
	Leading with constraints	"Given the recent budget cuts, what do we feel is most important to address first?"	
Positive assumptions	Focus on existing resources	"What are you already doing that is helpful, even just a little?" "What have you done in the past that helped?" "What would your colleagues say are your greatest strengths in this situation?"	Feel valued, trusted, respected.
	Use direct and indirect compliments	"I've noticed that you always approach your patients with so much compassion." "How did you manage to support the team given the challenges you were facing?"	Amplifies and reinforces strengths that team members may not be aware of; contributes to trust, respect, recognition, and autonomy.

healthcare leadership can be impersonal, hierarchical, and controlling (Suchman et al., 2011). The humanistic, solution-focused healthcare leader facilitates an organizational culture that supports the innate wholeness, strengths and resources, and self-actualization of staff, consistent with humanistic principles and enacted through solution-focused dialogue and skills. This enables leaders to lean into rather than avoid difficult conversations, as well as create conditions for their staff to do their best work.

In addition to promoting relationship-centred care, humanistic, solution-focused leadership also fosters a safety culture by supporting PS. Despite best intentions of hospital staff and leadership, 1 out of 17 hospital stays in Canada involves at least one harmful event such as medication errors, infections, and procedural complications (CIHI, 2022). Many of these safety events are preventable, and a proactive safety culture is the foundation to reducing preventable harm.

As the healthcare environment continues to evolve, so does the language for fostering a safety culture. Over the years, there has been a shift from traditional to proactive safety language in order to maximize PS and learning. Critical or blaming language can quickly put individuals on the defensive and discourages further dialogue and learning. On the other hand, a culture of PS promotes safety event reporting (Pfeifer, 2022) and is the foundation to achieving safer healthcare outcomes (Edmondson, 2017). From a solution-focused perspective, creating a psychologically safe environment supports frontline staff to share what is working and what is not, in order to drive meaningful and continuous process improvement. Safety events are often stressful experiences, and leaders can use strength-based (rather than deficit-based) communication strategies and tactics to help their teams navigate these challenging conversations. Shifting from critical language to solution-focused language helps to create the PS for staff to speak up about their experiences and ideas, and how work actually happens instead of how it's imagined. The dialogic strategies create opportunities to move away from path dependence, which is the tendency to keep doing things the way they've always been done before (Morgan & Barden, 2015), and instead move towards new solutions and innovation. Leaders can then guide the team to explore learnings from past successes to navigate similar situations (Berg & Szabo, 2005), and help teams imagine a preferred future in spite of existing constraints. Individuals and teams are encouraged to generate action steps for themselves based on existing assets as well as prior successes (Iveson et al., 2012). These communication strategies enhance dialogue, trust, and psychological safety, and ultimately improve safety for patients and employees (Edmondson, 2017).

Discussion

Adopting a humanistic, solution-focused leadership style addresses two of the most pressing issues in the current healthcare system: worker psychological well-being and psychological safety. Solution-focused leadership mindset shifts the paradigm and focus from "broken system" to "resources, strengths and possibilities," and effectively motivates teams to move forward despite the challenges they experience.

Leaders are optimally positioned and ultimately accountable to foster this possibility mindset, which is crucial for healthcare system sustainability. However, shifting the culture of a healthcare organization is difficult, *and* possible, and the resulting impact on staff experience and patient outcomes will be immeasurable. This process can be made easier with direct support from the senior leadership team. However, there is no need to wait for permission to adopt a solution-focused approach. Leadership can be practised by anyone, anywhere, whether it's a clinical manager, Human Resources associate, or front-line nurse.

Case Scenarios

Addressing employee mental health

In response to concerns about employees' well-being during the pandemic, a hospital appoints an employee mental health committee with representation from across the organization. The hospital has traditionally offered individual resources such as an Employee Assistance Program, health benefits, yoga, and mindfulness meditation classes. Clearly, more is needed at this time. The committee is tasked with figuring out what to do next.

SF leadership skill: Build a shared vision of the preferred future. *It's 5 years from now, and our hospital has addressed employee mental health so effectively that newspapers are writing about it.*

- *What do the headlines say?*
- *What are employees saying?*
- *Why do all the new grads want to work there?*
- *What strengths can we leverage?*
- *What's working right now?*
- *What can we do more of?*

Creating psychological safety to learn from patient safety incidents

A medication incident was identified on the unit. The patient identified that the medication given to them was the wrong dose. The pharmacy team was notified, and the staff involved felt a lot of stress, guilt, and shame as this could have led to significant harm if the error was not caught. The pharmacy manager is tasked with supporting the team through this incident and identifying improvement opportunities.

SF leadership skill: Nurture curiosity and learning. *I'm curious how you experienced this event. (Then pause, listen, and hold space for team member responses.)*

- *We made a mistake, **and** we are still a high performing team.*
- *This is a valuable learning opportunity for us all. When this type of error was caught in the past, what factors were at play?*

- *Given the challenges of increased interruptions to workflow, what could we try differently to protect team member attention and focus?*
- *When our medication processes are significantly safer in the future, what does that look like?*
- *What else?*
- *What strengths do we already have; what can we do more of?*
- *Who could we collaborate with for additional support in medication safety?*
- *What could we do differently to better support each other during this process?*

Grappling with change

The hospital you are working for is undergoing significant restructuring. The 12 Transition Navigators (TNs) – who used to each work individually for their respective departments – have been brought together as one centralized team. Each TN has different ways of doing things and different relationships with the teams they support. They are used to being in their own office, and now they are in one large room together. It's noisy. It's tense. How might you be able to support them?

SF leadership skill: Make the preferred future visible. *A year from now, when this team is working at its best:*

- *What will be happening?*
- *How will we be communicating with each other?*
- *What difference will that make?*
- *Who will notice? What impact would that have on them?*
- *What was helpful to achieving this vision?*
- *What else?*
- *What are the individual and collective strengths that we leveraged?*
- *What's one small change we could make now that could make a difference?*

Tackling workload stressors

Your team members have been complaining to you that the workload is unsustainable, with increased patient load, medical and psychosocial complexity, and being short staffed. People feel stretched, fatigued, and not in control of their workload. You noticed the quality of work is impacted and staff are looking to you for leadership and guidance. You also feel that the fatigue and the workload is taking a toll on you as well.

SF leadership skill: One foot in acknowledgement, one foot in possibility.

- *Take a pause; simply notice what thoughts and emotions are coming up for you in this scenario. See if you can acknowledge them without judgement towards yourself or others.*
- *On a scale of 10–1, where 10 is optimal functioning and 1 is the opposite, where would you say the team is at right now? Where are you right now?*
- *What makes it that number and not lower? What existing strengths are there for you and the team?*

- *Think of a moment in the past few weeks when things felt even just a little bit better. What was different?*
- *On days when it felt a little bit easier, what difference did that make?*
- *What would it take to make tomorrow or the next week 0.5–1 point higher on the scale?*
- *What steps would be even easier as a starting point?*
- *For the next week, notice the strengths you see in the team and try commenting out loud. Notice what difference that makes to you and the team.*

References

Bauserman, J. & Rule, W. (1995). *A Brief History of Systems Approaches in Counseling and Psychotherapy*. University Press of America, Inc.

Bayhan Karapinar, P., Metin Camgoz, S., & Tayfur Ekmekci, O. (2020). Employee wellbeing, workaholism, work–family conflict and instrumental spousal support: A moderated mediation model. *Journal of Happiness Studies, 21*(7), 2451–2471.

Berg, I.K. & Szabo, P. (2005). *Brief Coaching for Lasting Solutions*. Norton.

Boudrias, V., Trépanier, S.G., & Salin, D. (2021). A systematic review of research on the longitudinal consequences of workplace bullying and the mechanisms involved. *Aggression and Violent Behavior, 56*, article 101508.

Brown, C.L., Van Doren, N., Ford, B.Q., Mauss, I.B., Sze, J.W., & Levenson, R.W. (2020). Coherence between subjective experience and physiology in emotion: Individual differences and implications for well-being. *Emotion, 20*(5), 818–829.

Canadian Federation of Nurses Unions. (2022, February 2). Governments need to act now: Nurses are hanging on by a thread. Available at: https://nursesunions.ca/governments-need-to-act-now-nurses-are-hanging-on-by-a-thread/

Canadian Institute for Health Information (CIHI). (2022). Patient harm in Canadian hospitals? It does happen. Available at: https://www.cihi.ca/en/patient-harm-in-canadian-hospitals-it-does-happen

Canadian Medical Association. (2021). National physician health survey. Available at: https://www.cma.ca/physician-wellness-hub/content/physician-wellness-new-2021-national-physician-health-survey

Canadian Pharmacists Association. (2022). Pandemic stress, increase in harassment and staffing challenges exact heavy toll on pharmacy professionals. Available at: https://www.pharmacists.ca/news-events/news/pandemic-stress-increase-in-harassment-and-staffing-challenges-exact-heavy-toll-on-pharmacy-professionals/

Cook, E. (2020). *Exploring the Influence of a Solution-Focused Coaching Intervention on Coach Communication Skills and Athlete Self-Actualization: An Action Research Study*. Doctoral dissertation, University of Toronto (Canada).

Edmondson, A.C. (2017). Why is psychological safety so important in healthcare? Institute for Healthcare Improvement Open School. Available at: https://www.youtube.com/watch?v=LF1253YhEc8

Edmondson, A.C. (2018). *The Fearless Organization: Creating Psychological Safety in the Workplace for Learning, Innovation, and Growth*. John Wiley & Sons Ltd.

Grailey, K.E., Murray, E., Reader, T., & Brett, S.J. (2021). The presence and potential impact of psychological safety in the healthcare setting: an evidence synthesis. *BMC Health Services Research, 21*(1), 773.

Iveson, C., George, E., & Ratner, H. (2012). *Brief Coaching: A Solution Focused Approach*. Routledge.

Jun, J., Ojemeni, M.M., Kalamani, R., Tong, J., & Crecelius, M.L. (2021). Relationship between nurse burnout, patient and organizational outcomes: Systematic review. *International Journal of Nursing Studies, 119*, article 103933.

King, G. & Keenan, S. (2022). Solution-focused coaching for friendship in pediatric rehabilitation: A case study of goal attainment, client engagement, and coach stances. *Physical & Occupational Therapy in Pediatrics*, *42*(2), 154–171.

King, M. (2019). The neural correlates of well-being: A systematic review of the human neuroimaging and neuropsychological literature. *The Psychonomic Society*, *19*(3), 779–796.

Kingston, M.B., Dowell, P., Mossburg, S.E., Makkenchery, A., & Hough, K.R. (2022). Annual Perspective: Psychological Safety of Healthcare Staff. Agency for Healthcare Research and Quality. Available at: https://psnet.ahrq.gov/perspective/annual-perspective-psychological-safety-healthcare-staff

Lin, P.T., Vu, T.T., Nguyen, V.P., & We, Q. (2022). Self-determination theory and accountant employees' psychological wellbeing: The roles of positive affectivity and psychological safety. *Frontiers in Psychology*, *13*, article 870771.

Lucas, R.E., Diener, E., & Suh, E. (1996). Discriminant validity of well-being measures. *Journal of Personality and Social Psychology*, *71*(3), 616–628.

Maslow, A.H. (ed.). (1959). *New Knowledge in Human Values*. Harper.

McClintock, A.H. & Fainstad, T. (2022). Growth, engagement, and belonging in the clinical learning environment: The role of psychological safety and the work ahead. *Journal of General Internal Medicine*, *37*(9), 2291–2296.

Mental Health Commission of Canada (MHCC). (2018). National Standard of Canada for Psychological Health and Safety in the Workplace. Available at: https://www.mentalhealthcommission.ca/nationalstandard

Montano, D., Schleu, J.E., & Hüffmeier, J. (2023). A meta-analysis of the relative contribution of leadership styles to followers' mental health. *Journal of Leadership & Organizational Studies*, *30*(1), 90–107.

Morgan, A. & Barden, M. (2015). *A Beautiful Constraint: How to Transform Your Limitations into Advantages, and Why It's Everyone's Business*. John Wiley & Sons Ltd.

Nafstad, H.E. (2015). Historical, philosophical and epistemological perspectives. In: S. Joseph (ed.), *Positive Psychology in Practice: Promoting Human Flourishing in Work, Health, Education, and Everyday Life* (pp. 9–30). John Wiley & Sons Ltd.

Niinihuhta, M. & Häggman-Laitila, A. (2022). A systematic review of the relationships between nurse leaders' leadership styles and nurses' work-related well-being. *International Journal of Nursing Practice*, *28*(5), article e13040.

O'Donovan, R. & McAuliffe, E. (2020). A systematic review exploring the content and outcomes of interventions to improve psychological safety, speaking up and voice behaviour. *BMC Health Services Research*, *20*(1), 1–11.

Pfeifer, L. (2022). *Measuring Psychological Safety, High-Reliability (HRO) Perception and Safety Reporting Intentions among Pediatric Nurses*. Boston College.

Shain, M. (2010). The Shain reports on psychological safety in the workplace – a summary. Mental Health Commission of Canada. Available at: https://www.mentalhealthcommission.ca/wp-content/uploads/drupal/Workforce_Psychological_Safety_in_the_Workplace_ENG.pdf

SHCWEP. (2022). Survey on Health Care Workers' Experiences During the Pandemic: Detailed information for 2020 to 2021. Available at: https://www23.statcan.gc.ca/imdb/p2SV.pl?Function=getSurvey&SDDS=5362

Suchman, A., Sluyter, D., & Williamson P. (2011). *Leading Change in Healthcare: Transforming Organizations Using Complexity, Positive Psychology and Relationship-Centered Care*. Radcliffe Publishing Ltd.

UKG. (2023). *Mental Health at Work: Managers and Money*. The Workforce Institute. Available at: https://www.ukg.co.uk/resources/article/mental-health-work-managers-and-money

Umoren, R., Kim, S., Gray, M.M., Best, J.A., & Robins, L. (2022). Interprofessional model on speaking up behaviour in healthcare professionals: a qualitative study. *BMJ leader*, *6*(1), 15–

Wang, Y., Han, T., Han, G., & Zheng, Y. (2023). The relationship among nurse leaders' humanistic care behavior, nurses' professional identity, and psychological security. *American Journal of Health Behavior*, *47*(2), 321–336.

17 Humanistic, Solution-Focused Implementation

Organization and System Implications

Joanne Maxwell

At Holland Bloorview Kids Rehabilitation Hospital, our vision is to support the most meaningful and healthy futures for all children, youth, and families. In order to realize this vision, we need to support our clients and families to develop the skills, self-determination, and resiliency needed to successfully navigate life (healthcare, school, work, home, friends, and family).

Specific to their healthcare journey, our organization has a particular focus on supporting children, youth, and families through transitions that occur due to changes in services as a child develops. Through this organization-wide transitions strategy, which was launched in 2017, it was identified that we wanted to enhance staff capacity to facilitate client and family resiliency in the face of life challenges. We identified solution-focused coaching (SFC) as an approach that would support this goal and we embarked upon an organizational strategy to build capacity in SFC. As a healthcare leader, and one of the co-leads for this strategy, it is my privilege to share some of my thoughts on the impacts of this work at levels of the recipient of care (client and families), providers, leaders, and the organization. I will also speak to the evolution of the approach over time (to our current humanistic healthcare and education program), my own personal reflections and learnings as a leader, and the potential I see for system impact as we extend our reach well beyond the walls of our organization, to other healthcare organizations, and educational institutions.

What Initially Drew Us to SFC?

Our organization was compelled by the focus on strengths and the focus on the future that was evident in SF approaches. The origins of this future-focused, strengths-based approach, in solution-focused brief therapy, stemmed from a desire to shift from a focus on problems to a focus on solutions, with an emphasis on a future orientation in which client control and choice are inherent (Lloyd & Dallos, 2006). We also knew from our colleagues who had done some training in SF approaches that it is an approach that works well in coaching conversations (Ratner et al., 2012). The assumption of client strengths and competence allows us to place emphasis on noticing what is going well, something that is very powerful in a healthcare environment where the focus is so often on deficits and delays. The focus on strengths has been shown to support the development of new and novel ways to address problems (McAllister, 2003).

DOI: 10.4324/9781003414490-21

We were also drawn to the SF approach because it was something that could be broadly learned and adopted in our interprofessional context. It offered techniques that could be used by any member of the care team, and by the clients and families themselves. As we rolled out the education to our clinical staff, and then expanded it to our leaders, and then to family and youth leaders, we immediately noticed the positive impacts on engagement. This strengths-based, future-oriented, client- and family-centred approach to conversations allowed our teams to shape clinical conversations to the unique needs and wants of our clients and families. We began with a two-day initial training and offered additional sessions to reinforce learning and develop practical skills in SFC.

At the outset, as is nearly always the case with organizational change, the going was hard. We heard from clinicians that they felt "coaching" approaches didn't align with their clinical skills, and the focus on strengths was inconsistent with their requirement to assess the client and identify areas (problems or deficits) on which their interventions would focus. Many clinicians voiced concerns around how the SF approach diminished their unique professional contributions, and the open questions around "best hopes" left them without their usual control over the direction of the sessions. Others visibly bristled at the term "solution-focused" as it suggested there would always be a solution – and this was not their experience. These were valid reflections, and it was clear that we were proposing a more significant change in practice than I first realized. In some ways, this approach was completely consistent with our aims to deliver client- and family-centred care, and to engage and enable the kids and youth we serve, but it also represented a paradigm shift with regard to our traditional models of care.

Many initiatives start with a bang and fizzle out when there is the slightest of pushback. I was asked recently what it was about the SF approach that made me believe that this was something that we needed to commit so much energy to continuing. I reflect on the factors that contributed to my willingness to advocate for this approach and to fight for continued support financially past the original funding window, and to a scope well beyond that of our original initiative. Regarding the reasons why I have remained so committed to our work under what is now called the humanistic healthcare and education program, there are two buckets in which they fall: One reason is the real and potential positive benefits to clients, families, clinicians, and leaders (including myself). This is an accessible approach that can be used in many settings, in numerous contexts, and allows for compassionate, authentic, client- and family-centred care. The second reason is, without doubt, the passion of a small number of amazing people who have demonstrated a commitment not only to practising in this way at an individual level, but also to the transformative power of this approach and the importance of ensuring that we identify and leverage every opportunity to share this power with others. These champions have not only been the catalyst for change within our organization, but also the unexpected spread beyond our hospital, and the creation of a sustainable program model that is self-funding, incredibly efficient, and recognized for its excellence. These are the driving forces behind my continued commitment to our organizational leadership in this work.

Change Is Hard

And still, the change has not always been easy. As noted above, in addition to the many competing priorities and techniques and approaches offered and endorsed within an organization, we heard many reasons why some of our clinical staff did not want to adopt SF approaches or felt they could not use these strategies in their roles. In these moments of challenge and resistance, it was helpful to use many of the same strategies and principles that underlie the SF approach – to listen with curiosity to the challenges of working in healthcare, listen to understand the perceived barriers to change, and focus on the strengths and resources of the clinicians. In Lipchik's 2002 book, entitled *Beyond Technique*, the author states, "Therapists can't change clients: Clients have to change themselves" (p. 97). This quote recognizes that our work is relationship-based and involves the real and total humanity of both the client and the therapist. In the same way, our expert SF educators could not, and can not, "change the therapists." The therapists had to, and have to, change themselves. Our role was to listen, use the key words, recognize when they were already using approaches that were consistent with SFC, highlight and illustrate the power of the approach, and demonstrate how it can be used in diverse contexts so that SF language no longer felt like the square peg being forced into the round role of service delivery, and instead felt like a key to improved relationships, more engagement, and better outcomes.

We All Have to Change Ourselves

It was critical that our clinicians felt their unique skills, experience, and expertise were valued. We demonstrated how one could still assess, measure, and compare function against norms, and that these did not have to be incongruous with SF practices of considering the strengths and resources of the person. Rather than seeing these as opposing factors in creating a plan for treatment, strengths and resources are a means of amplifying the impact, supporting the client to articulate which functional gains are going to make the most difference, and who in their lives is going to be a resource to support their desired gains.

Another strategy to support our efforts was to demonstrate how SF approaches can have positive impacts on clinician well-being and decrease the prevalence of burnout. Authors such as Grant (2017) have shown that the ability to use solution-focused approaches can reduce stress and build resilience in healthcare providers. With so many challenges in healthcare, the ability to offer an approach to care that supported both client- and family-centred care and self-preservation was a powerful selling point. As our staff and teams recognized that by honouring the strengths of the clients, and acknowledging their level of readiness to engage, they saw and experienced the lifting of some of the overwhelming sense of responsibility they were carrying. When they could allow themselves to shift from quasi-saviour (with all the answers) to a coach who partners with their clients around a desired future, many more clinicians became converts to this humanistic approach.

I think our shift in terminology from SFC to humanistic healthcare was also an important point in our journey. I remember at the time being concerned that in shifting our language we might lose some of the momentum we had gained because SFC was such a familiar term within our context, but my concerns were overstated. In fact, the broader language of humanistic communication has allowed us to reach a broader audience, and healthcare (and education) is certainly ready for a renewed focus on humanism. Everyone, regardless of their clinical background, can see how improved communication skills that support understanding and engagement and create opportunities for agency can contribute to their effectiveness.

An Approach Beyond Care

As we slowly worked to address concerns and provide evidence of positive impact, more and more of our clinical staff have embraced elements of the approach. Even beyond the clinical context, we have seen SF strategies finding their way into other settings. I often hear people start meetings with a question around "best hopes," and leaders will quite naturally ask questions about what we are "already doing" to support our goals, or "what will be different" when we are successful. These phrases would likely have seemed a bit forced in the past, but they are now very much part of how we engage at a leadership level. We have overtly found ways to engage strengths-based, SF language into our performance review conversations (which we call "Momentum") and in many of the resources we share with other organizations, providers, and with our clients and families (e.g., the Transitions Guide, available at: https://hollandbloorview.ca/research-education/knowledge-translation-products/transitions-guide). Even more impactful is to see this language reflected in our organization's strategic plan, and to hear our Family Leaders use these skills in advocating for their needs.

As we grew our internal education program and sought opportunities for sustainability through the facilitation of sessions for external groups, we quickly found ourselves supporting other organizations across the country that wanted to bring this same kind of education to their teams. While we continue to have a significant cohort of internal staff who take our certificate program each year, we now have full cohorts from several other organizations, and are doing a significant amount of external training with partners outside of healthcare. The growth and tremendous positive feedback we have received from other organizations has been incredibly rewarding – and occasionally a little bit frustrating when we consider just how difficult it has been to get our own staff to adopt these practices. While our external partners are so grateful and appreciative of the skills they are learning, I feel that we are sometimes guilty of not fully appreciating our own expertise and take for granted our leadership in this work.

Our external programming has taken off exponentially since Dr Elaine Cook (one of the "champions" I mention above) took over the reigns of the program in 2018. At the time, we were offering our internal two-day program for all staff and doing a few sessions for external partners in the Toronto area. When Elaine came on board, she brought an energy, a passion, and a vision that was considerably bigger and bolder than our original model. Elaine soon developed the full certificate program (SFHCC) that has gifted us many SF practitioners at Holland Bloorview, and has also graduated coaches from across Canada. It is with great admiration for Elaine's skills and expertise that I can now reference additional certificate courses for educators and leaders well beyond our organizational walls.

This brings me to the Funnel of Optimal Functioning (FOF) (see Chapter 1). Not only has Elaine been able to drive incredible growth and expansion of our model, but she is also contributing to the field in truly significant ways. Through the FOF, Elaine has brought clarity and precision to our humanistic approach. Nearly all graduates in our SFHCC (and educator) certificate courses note the power of this visual model that translates neuroscience into a practical and usable tool to understand a person's readiness for change. The evolution of the FOF has been another important component of our success, and is something we expect to further validate and refine through research.

The Time for Compassion

As a leader in healthcare in 2024, I am reminded every day of the need for compassion. Compassion in the care that is delivered, compassion for those providing care, and compassion for those making small and large decisions about how healthcare is delivered at the levels of teams, programs, organizations, and systems. I mention above that the healthcare system (and many other contexts) is ripe for a renewed recognition of our humanity. The pandemic and other system pressures have elevated our awareness of burnout and stress, and we risk the health of not only our clients and families, but also our healthcare providers if we do not foster environments that recognize our individual and collective humanity and embrace every opportunity to bring compassion to our work and support the agency of others. I believe in, and strive every day, to demonstrate the qualities of a humanistic leader. I am not just a champion and organizational lead for this work, it has become a big part of who I am as a leader. It has wiggled its way into my heart and my mind, and for that, I am grateful.

In conclusion, I will share a few reflections of where I see the power of our SF humanistic model.

First – for clients and families:

I have heard stories of how a parent wells up with tears when asked about their child's strengths, when their only experiences of healthcare previously have focused on what is wrong.

I have heard stories of a father go from concern about medical complexity to lighting up with joy at sharing his disabled daughter's love of creating art.

I have been delighted to see former clients embrace SF language and articulate to providers how valuable it would have been to have had experienced these strategies during their youth. How much more engaged and respected they would have felt with regard to their care.

I have heard a parent express how she and her son successfully managed a difficult transition to a new school with the support of SF approaches.

For clinicians:

I have heard first-hand clinicians talk about how it has changed their practice, and lifted a burden that they never knew existed.

I have heard of clinicians who have been able remain in their careers when they thought they would have to retire or change industries.

I have listened as clinicians have spoken about recognizing that a family was in a place on the "funnel" at which they were not ready to engage. The clinician was able to shift their mindset from frustration to acceptance, and adjust strategies to meet them where they were at.

What it means for leaders:

I have had personal experience of the power of listening carefully for what is already working and focusing on an individual's strengths to manage through challenging situations.

I have seen the power of creating agency in a team by the simple use of words that elicit what we will notice when we are successful, or what has worked in the past.

I have seen colleagues thoughtfully probing and giving space to better understand an issue rather than leaping to propose a solution.

I hear people being thoughtful about the words they use and seeking ways to authentically engage others as partners.

These are just examples within Holland Bloorview. The feedback that our external partners have shared around the impact across healthcare, education, and leadership is equally impactful, and even more powerful when I consider the potential to positively impact others. I am convinced that healthcare needs to embrace SF humanistic approaches in care and leadership. I believe that the strategies are sufficiently flexible, adaptable, and accessible that they can be used in almost any context without the exorbitant costs of other transformative change.

Being thoughtful about our language is critical. For a long time, healthcare seemed to forget its roots in humanism and compassion, in favour of hierarchical models that focus on care as a transactional event between those who hold expertise (and power), and those who need their help. For all the advancements in science and care, the model has lost a critical focus on the relationship between care provider and the client and has managed to erode the agency of both parties.

I am optimistic that we can be better, and I believe SF approaches are an important lever for positive change that can be effectively implemented across contexts, settings, systems, and roles. These are cost-effective, impactful communication strategies and techniques in which every organization should invest – not only to support clinicians, but also for leaders, and for clients and families.

References

Grant, A. (2017). Coaching as evidence-based practice: The view through a multiple-perspective model of coaching research. In: T. Bachkirova, G. Spence, & D. Drake (eds), *The SAGE Handbook of Coaching* (pp. 62–84). SAGE Publishing.

Lipchik, E. (2002). *Beyond Technique in Solution-Focused Therapy: Working with Emotions and the Therapeutic Relationship*. Guilford Press.

Lloyd, H. & Dallos, R. (2006). Solution-focused brief therapy with families who have a child with intellectual disabilities: A description of the content of initial sessions and the processes. *Clinical Child Psychology & Psychiatry, 11*(3), 367–386.

McAllister, M. (2003). Doing practice differently: Solution-focused nursing. *Journal of Advanced Nursing, 41*(6), 528–535.

Ratner, H., George, E., & Iveson, C. (2012). *Solution Focused Brief Therapy: 100 Key Points and Techniques*. Routledge.

Index

Note: References to illustrations are in *italics*. References to tables are in **bold**.

tool 6; components 6; development 149;
holding space 118; model 5, 118,
149; mother and daughter example
72–4; personal narrative 118–19;
positive focus 132–3; in practice 8–9;
progressing through 83; table **7**

generative questions: solution-focused
conversation 118, 133
goal-setting 18, 123; and challenging
behaviour 82–3; collaborative 10, 24;
process 99, 100
"good enough" concept: bioethicist's
daily work 38; gift of 108; and project
timeframe 30, 32; recognition of 102,
106, 107, 108, 111–12; scaling questions
75; vs perfectionism 10
growing up: choices 36, 37

Hargreaves, Andy: Big Five Challenges
126
healing vs fixing 6, 18; checklist 79
healthcare: compassion in 149–50;
concerns about 3; contribution of
solution-focused approach (SFA) 34;
current medical paradigm 3; evidence-
based 14; humanistic approach vs deficit
focus 6; leaders 137; learners 4; positive
experiences 98–9
healthcare crisis: COVID-19 pandemic 8;
reports on 3
healthcare provider (HCP) 14
healthcare systems: advocacy 102;
drawbacks 98; evolution 89–90;
leadership styles in 137; as mechanized
systems 90; navigating 96–7, 106;
negative encounters 98; and person-
centred care 98–100; roles 35
healthcare workers: and COVID-19
pandemic 137
holding space: Funnel of Optimal
Functioning (FOF) 118
Holland Bloorview Kids Rehabilitation
Hospital (Canada) 3, 35, 38; Board-
Certified Behaviour Analysts (BCBAs)
53; certification program 117, 118,
119–20, 124; Child Life Specialists/
Child Youth Workers 53; Family as
Faculty 102, 104; Family Leader/Mentor
102, 106, 106–7, 117; Family Resource
Centre 106; Humanistic Solution-
Focused Health Care approach 148;
Inpatient Behaviour Team 53; Intake
Team 53; solution focused healthcare

approach 48; solution-focused coaching
(SFC) 145–6; vision 145; Youth
Facilitators 53
hospital staff: mental health 8
Humanism: principles 131–2
humanistic education and training:
keywords **10**
Humanistic Solution-Focused Health Care
approach 69; family role 96–7; Holland
Bloorview Kids Rehabilitation Hospital
148; and identity formation 95; personal
narrative 95, 96–100; and wholeness 95,
96, 99
Humanistic Solution-Focused
Health Care Coaching 50;
personal narrative 70

idea generation: and solution-focused
approach (SFA) 31
identity formation: and Humanistic
Solution-Focused Health Care approach
95
inflation 126
Institute for Patient and Family Centred
Care (IPFCC) 38, 39

James, Charles & Turner, Tana: *Towards
Race Equity in Education* 127
judges: solution-focused coaching (SFC)
for 123

keywords: humanistic education and
training **10**
Kushner, Rabbi Harold: on fear 127

labelling 32, 109, 132; for and against
95–6
leadership styles: in healthcare systems
137; and psychological well-being
(PW) 137; *see also* solution-focused
leadership
leading from behind 35, 60, 83, 103, 104,
139; advantages 39; and solution-
focused leadership 138
legal system: application of solution-
focused approach (SFA) 120–3
LGBTQ2S+ students 127, 129, 130
life coaching: stereotypes 116; *see also*
solution-focused coaching
Lightfoot, Gordon 115
Likert scale: Patient Activation Measure
(PAM) 17
listening 104; for understanding
80–1

Printed in the United States
by Baker & Taylor Publisher Services